Obstetric Dermatology

Arieh Ingber

Obstetric Dermatology

A Practical Guide

Foreword by Mark Lebwohl

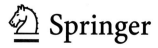 Springer

Professor Arieh Ingber
Clinical Associate Professor of Dermatology
Head, Department of Dermatology and Venereology
Hadassah University Hospital
Faculty of Medicine, Hebrew University
Jerusalem 91120
Israel

ISBN 978-3-642-10004-8   e-ISBN 978-3-540-88399-9

DOI: 10.1007/978-3-540-88399-9

Cover design: eStudio Calamar S.L.

Printed on acid-free paper

9 8 7 6 5 4 3 2 1

springer.com

To my wife, Tova, my children and my grandchildren.
A piece of evidence that I did something important when I wasn't
with them.

Foreword

There are many changes in the skin, hair, and nails during and after pregnancy. Patients are certainly aware that those changes are occurring, but few physicians and even fewer patients know how to predict the course of those changes. Pigmentary changes occur, but are they permanent? Can they be prevented or reversed? Hair may become thicker during pregnancy, only to fall out in the postpartum period. When will hair stop falling out? Will it grow back? What hormonal changes are occurring to produce these effects on the skin, hair, and nails? Will those hormonal changes affect other organs?

Some cutaneous manifestations of pregnancy are common and recognized by most physicians. Abdominal striae, for example, are easily identified, but physicians have many questions about them. Why do they develop? Can they be prevented or treated?

Other cutaneous manifestations of pregnancy are less common and recognized by few. For example, pruritic urticarial papules and plaques of pregnancy is a debilitating condition that is treatable once diagnosed. Even more important than the treatment, the knowledge imparted to a worried mother that her child will be fine and that the condition is self-limited is priceless; but the condition must first be recognized by the patient's physician.

All of these questions and conditions are addressed in this extraordinary book. Pigmentary disorders are addressed in detail in Chap. 2. Not only are readers told of the existence of disorders such as melasma, but the condition and its variable presentations are explained along with extensive discussion of the pathophysiology of the disorder as well an appropriately lengthy discussion of treatments. Disorders of hair and nails are covered extensively in Chap. 3, and all the questions raised in this foreword are answered well as are a multitude of other issues involving hair and nails during pregnancy. Chapter 1 offers a comprehensive review of hormonal changes in pregnancy that will serve students and residents in dermatology and obstetrics very well. These are elaborated on further in Chaps. 5 and 6, which discuss the physiologic changes caused by the hormonal alterations during pregnancy.

Much of the remainder of the book is devoted to specific pregnancy-related diseases. Each of these chapters combines a comprehensive review of the literature with clinical expertise that could only be written by a master clinician. The chapters on the various pruritic disorders of pregnancy could stand alone as classic references on a symptom complex that troubles many patients and their physicians. Undoubtedly, many patients will benefit from the information in this book, and many physicians will find answers to their perplexing questions about dermatologic disorders of pregnancy.

Some cutaneous manifestations of pregnancy are trivial and others are life-threatening to the mother and the fetus. The impact of pregnancy on diseases of the skin, and the impact of those diseases and their treatments on pregnancy are so varied and numerous that this subject is certainly worthy of a major textbook. Arieh Ingber has created a comprehensive work that will help obstetricians and dermatologists recognize and treat the many different conditions affecting the skin, hair, and nails during pregnancy. This should indeed become an important textbook for obstetricians, dermatologists, and students and residents.

Mark Lebwohl
The Sol and Clara Kest Professor of Dermatology
Chairman of Dermatology
The Mount Sinai School of Medicine

Preface

During pregnancy the skin may develop many changes: physiologic as well as pathologic. Most physicians are not familiar with these skin changes and have difficulty recognizing and diagnosing them correctly.

This book is a comprehensive overview guide for gynecologists, dermatologists, family physicians, and everyone who is interested in the appearance of the skin in pregnancy.

The information in this book is based on 30 years' experience of the author with pregnant women with skin conditions and on up-to-date literature.

I believe that this book will be the gold standard in the field of obstetrics and the skin.

Israel, 2008   **Arieh Ingber**

Contents

Endocrine and Immunologic Alterations During Pregnancy

1

1.1
Hormonal Changes

During pregnancy, women undergo dramatic hormonal changes, which encompass many of the endocrine organs, and not just the ovarian or placental derived hormones [24]. These changes have major effects on many of the alterations seen in the skin of pregnant women, and are probably the main stimulators of events during pregnancy. These changes are probably mediated by hormonal receptors, which can be found throughout the skin, its appendages, and vasculature [24].

From an endocrine point of view, pregnancy may be divided into two periods – the first period, or the "ovarian" period, is mainly dominated by the production of estrogen and progesterone from the corpus luteum. This phase lasts for 80–90 days after the last period. The second period, or the "placental" period, is dominated by steroid hormone production by the fetoplacental unit [11, 13, 18]. This interplay has been called "luteal placental shift" [13, 28].

The production of human chorionic gonadotropin (hCG) starts soon after nidation, leading to production of steroid hormones by the corpus luteum; hCG can be measured in blood as early as 48 h after implantation [11, 28]. The production of hCG by the placenta reaches a peak in the 12th week and then quickly declines by the 20th week, once estrogen and progesterone levels increase [13]. In contrast, the production of human placental lactogen by the trophoblast does not start until the seventh to eighth week of gestation [28].

Progesterone is the central hormone during the first part of pregnancy, and serves as a precursor for some fetal hormones [10]. During physiologic pregnancy, progesterone levels are 4–6 times higher than in nonpregnant women. Deoxicorticosterone, one of its metabolites, is found in concentrations 1,000 times higher than in nonpregnant women, but the physiologic role of this hormone is still not known [9].

During the first week of pregnancy, there is a gradual rise in progesterone levels, reaching a plateau or even a decrease in progesterone concentration during the seventh to tenth weeks of gestation. The reduction in progesterone levels can be relatively sharp and long-lasting in individual cases [28]. This pattern can be attributed to the gradual termi-nation of the corpus luteum and the following onset of placental progesterone produc-tion and secretion [20]. After that, progesterone levels continue to rise until delivery in uncomplicated pregnancies [28]. The corpus luteum has a major role in early pregnancy, and this has been demonstrated clinically by showing that its removal before the seventh or eighth week of gestation causes a decrease in serum progesterone concentration and leads to abortion [6, 22].

Estrogen levels start to rise shortly after implantation, with an additional rise at the sixth and seventh weeks of gestation, reflecting the takeover of estradiol production and secretion by the placenta [28]. Estrogen levels continue to rise during the second and third trimester until delivery [28]. Estrogen concentration reaches levels 3–8 times higher com-pared with levels in nonpregnant women [9]. Estrogen-level increase during pregnancy is the result of a unique transaction between mother and fetus. The fetus produces adrenal dehydroepiandrosterone and dehydroepiandrosterone sulfate by using the pregnenolone produced by the placenta. Thereafter, the placenta metabolizes these hormones to produce androstenedione. Lastly, they are transformed to estrone and estradiol and released into maternal circulation [9].

As stated previously, other endocrine organs change dramatically during pregnancy [24]. Along with a significant weight increase of the anterior pituitary gland (by more than twofold), there is an increased output of gonadotropins, corticotropin, ACTH, and melanocyte-stimulating hormone [14, 18]. Hypertrophy of the adrenal cortex can be seen along with increased production and secretion of hormones, including cortisol, aldoster-one, and dehydroepiandrosterone [24].

The thyroid gland also changes during pregnancy [24]. Hypertrophy of the thyroid gland can be seen as a result of a relative iodine deficiency during pregnancy. This leads to increased secretion of thyroid hormones in the second trimester, resulting in an increased basal metabolic rate [13, 24]. The parathyroid glands also hypertrophy, leading to a ten-dency toward low serum calcium levels [13]. This reduction in calcium levels may have an important role in the pathogenesis of impetigo herpetiformis during pregnancy [13].

1.2
Immunologic Changes

Pregnancy represents a unique and intriguing immunologic state, in which the maternal immune response is extensively altered to allow genetically different fetal tissues to attach to the mother without activating acute rejection [32]. These alterations are vital for the survival of the fetal allograft [8]. Owing to its important impact on potential understand-ing and treatment of organ transplantation rejection, this phenomenon has been immensely studied. Although many immunologic mechanisms have been found to be the cause of this phenomenon, they are still far from being completely understood [32].

Several studies suggest that cytokines produced by both T cells and non T cells play a critical role for fetal survival and growth [26]. For example, it was found that T-cell clones isolated from the deciduas of women with recurrent abortions produced significantly lower concentrations of IL-4 than clones derived from the deciduas of voluntary abortions or the endometrium of nonpregnant women [15]. The levels of monocytic IL-12 and TNF-α produced during the third trimester are lower than the postpartum values [15]. Th2 cytokines, such as IL-10, have been found at higher levels in the placenta and amniotic fluid during the third trimester of pregnancy [12], and IL-6 serum levels steadily increase in maternal circulation and even more during labor [3]. TNF-α serum levels do not vary during pregnancy; however, TNF-α soluble receptor levels increase, thus helping to protect the fetus from the deleterious effects of TNF-α [16].

The cytokine complex is a very complicated and sophisticated one; however, overall, it is thought that during pregnancy there is a tendency toward the Th2 cytokines (IL-4, IL-10, etc.), which favor the maintenance of fetal survival [26]. The levels of Th1 cytokines (IL-2, interferons, TNF-α) are elevated in the early postpartum period [26]. As will be described later in this book, women with Th1-mediated cytokine diseases, such as rheumatoid arthritis, psoriasis, and multiple sclerosis, frequently get better during pregnancy, only for these diseases to be exacerbated, or present, in the postpartum period [26].

The cellular immune system also undergoes major changes. For example, the absolute numbers of CD3, CD4, CD8, and CD20 cells decrease during pregnancy and the numbers of CD4, CD20, and CD16 cells increase 1 month postpartum and those of CD3 and CD56 cells increase at 4 months postpartum [23].

Humoral immunity is also significantly affected during pregnancy [17]. In pregnancy, there is an increased production of asymmetric IgG antibodies [30]. In addition, pregnancy-specific glycoproteins (PSG), namely, PSG1, PSG6, PSG6N, and PSG11, have been found to induce the secretion of the anti-inflammatory cytokines IL-10, IL-6, and TGF-β$_1$ in vitro, but not of IL-1β, TNF-α or IL-12 [29].

Human leukocyte antigen G is a nonclassic major histocompatability complex molecule (class Ib), the expression of which at the fetal–maternal boundary has been implicated in maternal tolerance during pregnancy [32]. This major histocompatability complex molecule interacts with inhibitory leukocyte immunoglobulin like receptors 1 and 2, and natural killer cell receptors, thus modulating immune function [1, 4, 5].

As described in the first part of this book, pregnancy is accompanied by major changes in endocrine function. There is a major research effort to elucidate the interactions of pregnancy-related hormones and the immune system [26]. The in vitro secretion of numerous cytokines is inhibited by estrogen [19]; estrogen suppresses IL-2 production at the transcriptional level, accompanied by inhibition of IL-2 receptor (IL-2R) expression by 17β-estradiol [31]. At physiologic concentrations, progesterone promotes the production of Th2 cytokines IL-4 and IL-5, and leads to production of the progesterone-induced blocking factor by the lymphocytes, a mediator protein which induces a Th2-biased immune response [2]. At pharmacologic levels, such as those observed during the second part of pregnancy, progesterone has an inhibitory effect on TNF-α secretion and a stimulatory effect on IL-10 synthesis in T-lymphocyte clones, leading to an increased humoral immune response [7].

Glucocorticoid levels increase steadily during pregnancy [2]. Glucocorticoids are a well-known immunosuppressive agent, which act by inhibiting IL-1, TNF-α, interferon-γ, and IL-2 production and by stimulating IL-10, IL-4, and IL-13 synthesis [25]. Other hormones such as prolactin, human-placental lactogen, and hCG can have significant immunosuppressive effects similar to those found in pregnancy at high levels [2].

Overall, the physiologic increase of cortisol, progesterone, estradiol, and testosterone levels during the third trimester of pregnancy seems to lead to Th2 cytokine preference both at the systemic level and at the fetal–maternal interface [21, 27].

Summary

> During pregnancy women undergo dramatic hormonal changes, encompassing all the major endocrine organs.
> During the first trimester pregnancy is hormonally maintained by the corpus luteum, and later the placenta takes over. Progesterone is the central hormone during the first part of pregnancy, and except for a decline during the sixth to tenth weeks, its levels rise constantly. Estrogen levels continue to rise throughout pregnancy.
> Other major hormones modulated in pregnancy include the pituitary hormones, the adrenal hormones, and the thyroid and parathyroid hormones.
> During pregnancy the maternal immune response is extensively altered to allow the fetus to attach to the mother. Several immunologic alterations have been found in many of the immunologic mechanisms.
> Cytokine profile is altered, leading overall to a tendency toward the Th2 cytokines, which favor the maintenance of fetal survival. Postpartum there is elevation in the levels of Th1 cytokines.
> The cellular immune system undergoes major changes, as well as humoral immunity. In addition, the expression of human leukocyte antigen G at the fetal–maternal boundary leads to maternal tolerance during pregnancy.
> Hormonal changes during pregnancy lead overall to preference of the Th2 cytokine profile.

References

1. Allan DS, Lepin EJ, Braud VM et al (2002) Tetrameric complexes of HLA-E, HLA-F, and HLA-G. J Immunol Methods 268:43–50
2. Ansar Ahmed S, Penhale WJ, Talal N (1985) Sex hormones, immune responses, and autoimmune diseases. Mechanisms of sex hormone action. Am J Pathol 121:531–551
3. Branch DW (1992) Physiologic adaptations of pregnancy. Am J Reprod Immunol 28:120–122
4. Clements CS, Kjer-Nielsen L, Kostenko L et al (2005) Crystal structure of HLA-G: a nonclassical MHC class I molecule expressed at the fetal-maternal interface. Proc Natl Acad Sci USA 102:3360–3365
5. Colonna M, Samaridis J, Cella M et al (1998) Human myelomonocytic cells express an inhibitory receptor for classical and nonclassical MHC class I molecules. J Immunol 160:3096–3100
6. Csapo AI, Pulkkinen MO, Ruttner B et al (1972). The significance of the human corpus luteum in pregnancy maintenance. I. Preliminary studies. Am J Obstet Gynecol 112:1061–1067
7. Cutolo M, Sulli A, Seriolo B et al (1995) Estrogens, the immune response and autoimmunity. Clin Exp Rheumatol 13:217–226
8. Davison SC, Ballsdon A, Allen MH et al (2001) Early migration of cutaneous lymphocyte-associated antigen (CLA) positive T cells into evolving psoriatic plaques. Exp Dermatol 10:280–285

9. Doria A, Iaccarino L, Sarzi-Puttini P et al (2006) Estrogens in pregnancy and systemic lupus erythematosus. Ann N Y Acad Sci 1069:247–256

10. Doria A, Iaccarino L, Arienti S et al (2006) Th2 immune deviation induced by pregnancy: the two faces of autoimmune rheumatic diseases. Reprod Toxicol 22:234–241

11. Elling SV, Powell FC (1997) Physiological changes in the skin during pregnancy. Clin Dermatol 15:35–43

12. Greig PC, Herbert WN, Robinette BL et al (1995) Amniotic fluid interleukin-10 concentrations increase through pregnancy and are elevated in patients with preterm labor associated with intrauterine infection. Am J Obstet Gynecol 173:1223–1227

13. Hellreich P (1974) The skin changes of pregnancy. Cutis 13:82–86

14. Hill B (1953) The skin and its normal and abnormal states in pregnancy. N Z J Med 53:151–156

15. Iwatani Y, Amino N, Tachi J et al (1988) Changes of lymphocyte subsets in normal pregnant and postpartum women: postpartum increase in NK/K (Leu 7) cells. Am J Reprod Immunol Microbiol 18:52–55

16. Kupferminc MJ, Peaceman AM, Aderka D et al (1995) Soluble tumor necrosis factor receptors in maternal plasma and second-trimester amniotic fluid. Am J Obstet Gynecol 173:900–905

17. Margni RA, Zenclussen AC (2001) During pregnancy, in the context of a Th2-type cytokine profile, serum IL-6 levels might condition the quality of the synthesized antibodies. Am J Reprod Immunol 46:181–187

18. McKenzie AW (1971) Skin disorders in pregnancy. Practitioner 206:773–780

19. McMurray RW, Ndebele K, Hardy KJ et al (2001) 17-beta-estradiol suppresses IL-2 and IL-2 receptor. Cytokine 14:324–333

20. Mishell DR Jr, Thorneycroft IH, Nagata Y et al (1973) Serum gonadotropin and steroid patterns in early human gestation. Am J Obstet Gynecol 117:631–642

21. Munoz-Valle JF, Vazquez-Del Mercado M, Garcia-Iglesias T et al (2003) T(H)1/T(H)2 cytokine profile, metalloprotease-9 activity and hormonal status in pregnant rheumatoid arthritis and systemic lupus erythematosus patients. Clin Exp Immunol 131:377–384

22. Murthy YS, Arronet GH, Parekh MC (1970) Luteal phase inadequacy. Its significance in infertility. Obstet Gynecol 36:758–761

23. Narita M, Yamada S, Kikuta H et al (2000) Reconstitution of humoral immunity during pregnancy. Am J Reprod Immunol 44:148–152

24. Nussbaum R, Benedetto AV (2006) Cosmetic aspects of pregnancy. Clin Dermatol 24:133–141

25. Ramirez F, Fowell DJ, Puklavec M et al (1996) Glucocorticoids promote a TH2 cytokine response by CD4+ T cells in vitro. J Immunol 156:2406–2412

26. Raychaudhuri SP, Navare T, Gross J et al (2003) Clinical course of psoriasis during pregnancy. Int J Dermatol 42:518–520

27. Salem ML (2004) Estrogen, a double-edged sword: modulation of TH1- and TH2-mediated inflammations by differential regulation of TH1/TH2 cytokine production. Curr Drug Targets Inflamm Allergy 3:97–104

28. Schindler AE (2005) Endocrinology of pregnancy: consequences for the diagnosis and treatment of pregnancy disorders. J Steroid Biochem Mol Biol 97:386–388

29. Schuurs AH, Verheul HA (1990) Effects of gender and sex steroids on the immune response. J Steroid Biochem 35:157–172

30. Snyder SK, Wessner DH, Wessells JL et al (2001) Pregnancy-specific glycoproteins function as immunomodulators by inducing secretion of IL-10, IL-6 and TGF-beta1 by human monocytes. Am J Reprod Immunol 45:205–216

31. Szekeres-Bartho J, Barakonyi A, Par G et al (2001) Progesterone as an immunomodulatory molecule. Int Immunopharmacol 1:1037–1048

32. Yip L, McCluskey J, Sinclair R (2006) Immunological aspects of pregnancy. Clin Dermatol 24:84–87

Hyperpigmentation and Melasma

2

2.1
Hyperpigmentation

Almost all women, presumably up to 90%, and particularly those with dark hair and complexions, note some degree of hyperpigmentation during pregnancy. Patients are often deeply concerned by this condition, and may view these changes with uneasiness, yet hardly ever do they voluntarily express their concerns [21].

There is usually a mild generalized pigmentation, most marked in areas that are already slightly darker than surrounding skin, such as the nipples, areola, neck, upper back, periumbilical skin, and midline of the abdomen (Figs. 2.1–2.3). Other areas that may perceptibly darken are areas of friction such as the medial thighs, the perineum, and the axillae. In addition, freckles, nevi, and recent scars may darken and even enlarge during gestation [1]. Generalized hypermelanosis may rarely develop, and its occurrence suggests hyperthyroidism [11].

In general, hyperpigmentation begins early in pregnancy, and is considered to be one of the earliest signs of pregnancy [5]. This condition progresses until delivery [40]. The areas of hyperpigmentation almost always lighten after delivery [7], but the affected sites usually do not return to their previous color [11].

There are special areas of hyperpigmentation which deserve special attention:

> Darkening of the skin adjoining the areolae produces what are called secondary areolae [39]. This areolar pigmentation should be differentiated from nevoid hyperkeratosis of the nipple and areola, a rare condition that has been reported to develop during pregnancy or even at puberty. Nevoid hyperkeratosis of the nipple and areola is reflected histologically by rete ridge elongation, papillomatosis, and hyperkeratosis with greatly dilated keratin-filled spaces [21].
> The linea alba ("white line"), the tendinous medial line on the anterior abdominal wall, turns dark to become the linea nigra, on the midline of the abdomen from the

A. Ingber, *Obstetric Dermatology*,
DOI: 10.1007/978-3-540-88399-9, © Springer-Verlag Berlin Heidelberg 2009

umbilicus to the symphysis pubis (Fig. 2.4). It can extend superiorly to the xiphoid process. It appears during the first trimester of pregnancy and, like other areas of hyperpigmentation, is most pronounced in dark-haired, dark-complexioned women [40]. This condition is often accompanied by displacement of the umbilicus, at term, to the right side of the patient, the "ligamentum teres" sign. This shift persists postpartum until the abdominal muscles regain their normal tone [21]. This displacement is the consequence of the pressure of the uterus on the ligamentum teres and falciform ligament [2]. The development of a darker areola and a linea nigra were used clinically in the past to establish parity [27].

 › Group B natural pigmentary demarcation lines have been reported to occur on the lower limbs during pregnancy. Pigmentary demarcation lines are borders of abrupt transition between more deeply pigmented skin and that of lighter pigmentation. One report describes two women developing demarcation lines: one developed the condition during her pregnancy, and the condition remained unchanged 8 months postpartum; the other developed the condition immediately postpartum [12]. Another report describes four cases of women developing demarcation lines; all of them developed the condition only during pregnancy, and it disappeared completely between the first and third months postpartum [37]. There were also reports of demarcation lines during pregnancy which were accompanied by erythema. While the erythema disappeared quickly, the pigmentation subsided more slowly. The explanation suggestion for this phenomenon was compression of peripheral nerves by the enlarged uterus in the late period of pregnancy, thus influencing the innervated cutaneous microvasculature to induce neurogenic inflammation with resultant erythema and pigmentation [26]. Demarcation lines were also reported to occur during pregnancy on the medial aspect of the arms [15].

 › Longitudinal melanonychia, which is commonly seen in black persons and orientals, but is rarely present in white women, was reported to develop in a white woman during pregnancy [9, 21].

 › Dermal melanocytosis is a rare dermatosis, which was found to darken during pregnancy. This dermatosis may also be triggered during pregnancy [31]. Reactivation of preexisting dormant dermal melanocytes by a variety of hormonal factors is thought to occur. Elevation in estrogen and progesterone levels and elevation in keratinocyte-derived endothelin 1 and melanocyte simulating hormone (MSH) levels upon sun exposure potentiate tyrosinase activity and thus stimulate melanogenesis [21].

2.2
Melasma

The term "melasma," or facial hyperpigmentation, is derived from the Greek *melas*, meaning "black" [8]. It has been also termed "chloasma gravidarum" and "the mask of pregnancy" [38] (Fig. 2.5). Its onset is usually during the second half of the gestational period, and it occurs in 45–75% of pregnancies [1, 11, 38]. It is said to be more common in dark-haired, brown-eyed, dark-complexion women [38, 40]. A review of major studies evaluating

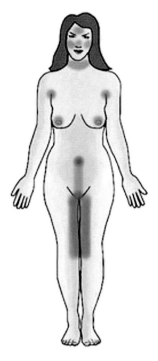

Fig. 2.1 Areas of hyperpigmentation

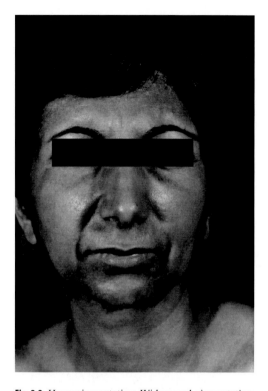

Fig. 2.2 Hyperpigmentation. Widespread pigmentation of the face in a dark-skinned pregnant women

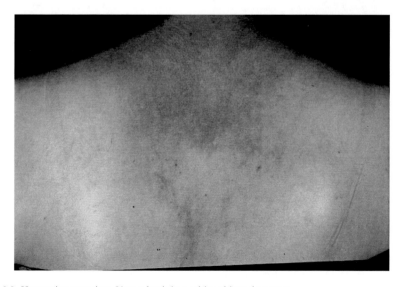

Fig. 2.3 Hyperpigmentation. Upper back in a white-skinned woman

2

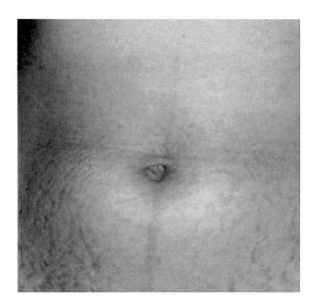

Fig. 2.4 Linea nigra on the middle part of the abdomen. Note also striae distensae

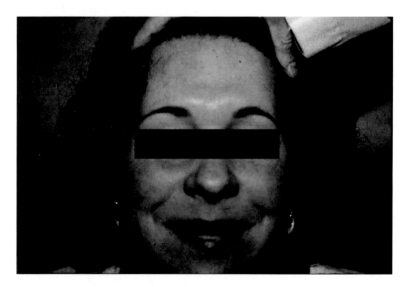

Fig. 2.5 Melasma. "The mask of pregnancy." Typical pigmentation on the cheeks and forehead

the incidence of melasma during pregnancy is summarized in Table 2.1. The major differences in the incidence of melasma in the different studies were attributed to the fact that pigmentary changes are more discernible in fair-skinned individuals [16].

Superimposed on the general pigmentation induced by pregnancy, melasma may appear as blotchy, irregular, sharply demarcated, tan to dark brown plaques or patches of pigmentation in symmetrical distribution on the forehead, temples, cheeks, and central areas of the

Table 2.1 Incidence of melasma according to major studies

No. of cases	Percentage of cases	References
65	46.40	[23]
10	8.50	[29]
15	2.50	[16]

face [11, 20, 38]. Less often, the perioral and mental areas are involved [38]. The number of hyperpigmented lesions may range from one single lesion to multiple patches [13].

Melasma may occur in three clinical patterns [32]:

> The centrofacial pattern – involves the cheeks, forehead, upper lip, nose, and chin. This pattern is observed in the majority of patients (63%).
> The malar pattern – hyperpigmentation localized to the cheeks and nose. This pattern was seen in 21% of patients.
> The mandibular pattern – involves the ramus of the mandible. This pattern comprised 16% of patients.

In none of these variants are the mucous membranes involved [5].

Basically, two patterns of pigmentation are observed histopathologically [32]:

> *Epidermal type*. The predominant site of melanin deposition is in the basal and suprabasal layers, and, occasionally, throughout the prickle layers up to the stratum corneum.
> *Dermal type*. This is characterized by the presence of melanin-laden macrophages in a perivascular array, both in the superficial and deep dermis.

There is normal epidermal thickness, but the number of melanocytes is thought to be increased [5, 21].

On the basis of both visible light and Wood's light examination, Sanchez et al. [32] have classified melasma into four major types:

> *Epidermal type*. Exhibits enhancement of color contrast when examined with Wood's light. When examined with natural light, this type will appear light brown.
> *Dermal type*. Exhibits no enhancement of color contrast when examined with Wood's light. When examined with natural light, this type will appear blue-gray.
> *Mixed type*. Wood's light examination reveals both enhancement of lesions in some areas and no enhancement of lesions in other areas. When examined with natural light, this type will appear deep brown
> *Wood's light inapparent*. Clinically apparent lesions after examination with visible light, but these lesions are not apparent with Wood's light examination. This pattern occurs in very dark individuals in whom the abnormally pigmented skin is close in color to the adjacent normal skin and pigment deposition is primarily dermal.

There is no correlation between the three clinical patterns of melasma and either the histopathologic examination or the Wood's light skin appearance [32].

Oral contraceptives are also a main etiologic factor of melasma, and melasma and pigmentation represent the most common cutaneous side effects of oral contraceptives: 5–34% of individuals are affected, the higher incidence being seen in the more deeply pigmented race. Hyperpigmentation of the face also occurs in some women during normal menstrual periods. Melasma during pregnancy indicates susceptibility to increased pigmentation with the contraceptive pill and the drug may induce melasma when none existed in pregnancy [20, 38]. Melasma during menstrual periods and melasma induced by the contraceptive pill may be predictive of women who will have pigmentary changes during pregnancy [38].

The etiologic factors in melasma include, other than pregnancy and oral contraception, the following [32]:

> *Cosmetics.* In the past, cosmetics made of poorly refined ingredients, containing irritating or phosphosensitizing substances, and increased occupational exposure to crude tars and oils were a major cause for melanosis of the face. Other ingredients in cosmetics that were selectively implicated as causative factors for dermal melanoses include certain fatty acids, photoactive contaminants of mineral oils, petrolatum, beeswax, certain dyes, *para*-phenylenediamine, and perfume ingredients.

> *Genetic and racial predisposition.* A genetic predisposition has been supported only by occasional reports of familial occurrence. There is a high occurrence of melasma in patients of Hispanic origin.

> *Medications.* A wide variety of medications have produced hyperpigmentation. These include metals such as arsenic, iron, copper, bismuth, silver, and gold and phototoxic and antiseizure drugs [5]. Hyperpigmentation has also followed the administration of organic compounds such as quinacrine and 5-ethyl-3-methyl-5-phenylhydantoin.

Other etiologic factors for the development of melasma are nutrition, liver disease, and parasitosis [5, 8]. A significant association was also found in nonpregnant women between thyroid autoimmunity and melasma, primarily in women whose condition developed during pregnancy or after the ingestion of oral contraceptive drugs [10].

Exposure to UV light radiation plays a significant etiologic role in the pathogenesis of melasma, and is felt to be necessary for the development of melasma [8]. The majority of patients with melasma observed the onset of their melasma during the summer months. Sun exposure is also a prominent cause of exacerbation of melasma, while during the winter months, melasma appears to be less noticeable [32]. The areas of the face that are most affected are those that have maximum exposure to the sun. Clearly, however, many women are exposed to sunlight during pregnancy without developing melasma [40].

In a study of 210 melasma patients, the incidence of various causative factors was found to be universally due to sunlight exposure (100%), and in descending order was due to pregnancy (27%), cosmetics (14%), familial factors (13%), and oral contraceptive use (6.3%) [13].

The course of melasma is progressive during pregnancy [38], but its intensity is not necessarily proportional to that of general melanosis. Unlike the persistent melasma associated with the use of oral contraceptives, the melasma of pregnancy usually fades within 1 year of delivery, but it may occasionally persist if the hyperpigmentation is deep

[11, 20, 38]. The persistence incidence was reported to be less than 10%, although one study found persistence in 30% of cases after 10 years [1, 40]. If it is persistent postpartum, some women note a premenstrual hyperpigmented flare [5].

2.3
Pathogenesis of Pigmentation

The enzyme responsible for melanin production is tyrosinase, a copper-containing oxygenase enzyme, which mediates melanin production through the intermediate, L-dopa [27]. Tyrosinase activity may be regulated by many factors. For example, incubation of human melanocytes with 1,25-dihydroxyvitamin D_3, α-MSH, and β-estradiol caused an increase in tyrosinase activity [30]. Nevertheless, no specific receptors have yet been demonstrated on the melanocyte [27].

Hyperpigmentation in pregnancy is attributed by some investigators to an increased output of some combination of placental, pituitary, and ovarian hormones [40]. An increased amount of MSH of the pituitary was postulated in the past to be the cause of hyperpigmentation. It was even believed that the demonstration of MSH in urine could be used as a pregnancy test [4].

Shizume and Lerner [33] showed by analyzing the urine of 38 pregnant and postpartum women and the blood of 13 pregnant women using bioassay methods that after the second month of pregnancy MSH levels in the urine became elevated above normal levels. MSH levels continued to increase until delivery, and then rapidly decreased to normal within 5 days postpartum. The importance of MSH in pregnancy was also suggested by other investigators [4, 19].

Later, these bioassay methods were doubted, because they lacked real specificity; it has not been possible to identify the substances and it was not clear if they were of pituitary origin [36].

Since the major pituitary MSH in the human is thought to be β-MSH, Thody et al. [36] measured plasma β-MSH levels in pregnancy and postpartum using a specific radioimmunoassay. They showed that plasma β-MSH levels in late pregnancy were within the normal range and were no different from the levels in women after parturition.

Later, the levels of circulating immunoreactive α-MSH were evaluated during pregnancy. It was found that during the first trimester immunoreactive α-MSH levels were undetectable in plasma of most subjects. During late pregnancy, however, the levels of α-MSH were significantly higher than those of the control. It was concluded that α-MSH has no pigmentary role in pregnancy because the pigmentation begins early and is normally focal, unlike that of Addison's disease and Cushing's syndrome [3].

Other factors which were suggested to be related to hyperpigmentation in pregnancy are progesterone and estrogen, the levels of both of which are increased during pregnancy [7]. Blood levels of progesterone increase throughout pregnancy, and estrogen production rises from the eighth week and begins to decrease after the 30th week of pregnancy. This pattern follows the progression of hyperpigmentation [18]. Using guinea pigs as a model and by utilizing controlled histochemical experiments, Snell et al. [34] showed that estrogen, when given alone in small doses, increased the output of melanin by the melanocytes and exerted its greatest influence on sexual skin – the areola. When the dose was raised, the effect was increased and was accompanied by a rise in the melanocyte count in the skin of the anterior abdominal wall. The effect of small doses of estrogen was shown to be augmented by giving progesterone at the same time. These hormones were thus suggested to be strong stimulants of melanogenesis.

Thus, hyperpigmentation of the face occurs in women taking oral contraceptives or during the menstrual cycle, supporting the idea that estrogen and progesterone are involved [27]. In addition, hyperpigmentation of the face is associated with disorders involving the function of the uterus and ovaries, a condition termed "chloasma uterinum" [24].

A small study found that nevi from patients who are pregnant or 1 month postpartum have increased numbers of estrogen and progesterone binding sites. The time of onset of increased hormonal binding of nevi in pregnancy could not be determined in this study, but it was speculated to be prior to 5 months' gestation [6].

It should be noted that although progesterone, estrogen, and MSH were implicated as causative factors in melasma of pregnancy, they have not been found to be consistently elevated in melasma in general [32]. Generally, the hormone levels with oral contraceptives are not though to be high enough to initiate melasma [22]. A study evaluating MSH levels in nine women with idiopathic melasma (nonpregnancy or oral-contraceptive-associated melasma) found no elevation of MSH levels compared with levels in controls [28].

Recently, investigators found that a lipid extraction from the placenta had a pigment-inducing activity both in vivo and in vitro. The placenta was found to be rich in bioactive sphingolipids, which were found to induce melanogenesis by upregulating the expression of various melanogenic enzymes – tyrosinase and tyrosinase-related proteins 1 and 2 at the translational and transcriptional levels [17].

Wade et al. [38] have suggested that the reason why only certain body areas, but not the entire body, are affected by hyperpigmentation is that melanocytes in the areas affected are more sensitive to hormonal stimulation. Another explanation may be the greater population of melanocytes in the affected sites [40]. One investigation showed that there is a greater population of melanocytes in the skin of the face and forehead, with the population density of melanocytes being 2–4 times greater than in the skin of the thigh and arms [35].

2.4
Treatment

Treatment of pigmentary alteration in pregnancy is unsatisfactory and preventive measures or treatment for hyperpigmentation in pregnancy is limited [40]. For generalized hyperpigmentation, many physicians do not recommend therapy other than sunscreens for sun-exposed areas [41].

The treatment of melasma is usually postponed until after delivery for apparent reasons: (1) the hormonal cause for melasma persists throughout pregnancy, making melasma more resistant to treatment; (2) most women have a significant improvement in melasma after parturition, making therapy unnecessary; (3) the mainstay of therapy for melasma is relatively contraindicated during pregnancy [25].

During pregnancy, women should avoid heavy suntanning and should use broad-spectrum (UVA and UVB) sunscreens and appropriate clothing [22, 40]. In addition, patients are encouraged to use opaque sunscreens to diminish all UV and visible light in order to minimize further pigment production [22]. It has been demonstrated that a correlation exists between the use of sunscreen and the result of melasma treatment [13]. Sunbathing is absolutely contraindicated, as a few minutes of sunbathing can reverse the benefit of months of therapy [13].

Avoidance of trauma, especially if the patient is prone to easy scarring (scars may hyperpigment) is recommended, and patients are cautioned to avoid rubbing or irritation [22]. Cosmetics on the face, especially perfumed preparations, should be avoided; however, the patients may choose to use nonallergenic, skin-colored, cover-up preparations. Nonhormonal methods of contraception should be considered.

Bleaching agents have been used with variable, but usually poor, results. Phenolic compounds were regarded as dangerous as they can cause considerable skin irritation, contact dermatitis, and dyschromias. However, two trials have shown satisfactory results without major side effects. The combination of 4-hydroxianisol (2%) and tretinoin (0.01%) and the use of n-acetyl-4-S-cysteaminylphenol in a 4% oil-in-water emulsion applied twice daily for 6 months were found to give good results [13]. Vitamin C was used systematically in mild forms of melasma, and vitamin E seems to act synergistically to vitamin C.

A report by Kligman and Willis [14] shows satisfactory results in 14 of 16 patients with melasma using a formulation of tretinoin (0.1%), hydroquinone (5%), and dexamethasone (0.1%). The vehicle was hydrophilic ointment or a solution of equal parts of ethanol and propylene glycol. The patients in this study were young, adult, white women taking contraceptive pills. The regimen used was once-daily application. The depigmentation was of satisfactory magnitude by 5–7 weeks after the start of the treatment. No adverse effects were reported, and normal skin was only slightly, if at all, lightened.

The usefulness of depigmenting agents is dependent on the histologic classification and Wood's light typing described by Sanchez et al. [32]. The predominantly epidermal type of melasma responds to formulations containing 2% hydroquinone plus 0.05% retinoic acid with nightly use. Melasma of mixed type with predominantly dermal deposition of melanin, however, responds poorly to this therapy [32]. Wong and Ellis [40] reported that their experience with 2–5% hydroquinone is only partially effective in some patients with the epidermal type of melasma, even after months of use.

A slight modification to the treatment suggested by Kligman and Willis was reported by Katsambas and Antoniou [13]. Their formulation includes 4% hydroquinone, 0.05% tretinoin, and 1%hydrocortisone acetate, which is applied twice a day until patients reach the desired degree of depigmentation, but never for more than 8–10 weeks [13]. Another treatment suggestion is the use of 0.05% tretinoin, 2% hydroquinone, and 0.1% bethamethasone valerate cream [13].

Hydroquinone is in the US FDA pregnancy category C because studies have never been conducted to see whether hydroquinone causes fetal harm when applied topically [25]. Tretinoin is in US FDA pregnancy category C and in category D in the equivalent Australian administration. There are several reports of fetal malformation when mothers used tretinoin during pregnancy; nonetheless, causation cannot be definitely determined [25].

The development of hypopigmented lesions is a potential side effect of the treatment with the combinations described above, but the risk can be minimized with proper patient education and follow-up examination [39]. Other side effects include dermatitis and hyperpigmentation [40]. In addition, the prolonged and excessive use of preparations of hydroquinone higher than 3% can result in ochronosis, a blue-black postinflammatory discoloration [13].

Azelaic acid cream has been reported to be of benefit in the treatment of melasma when applied twice daily. Various study have shown good to excellent results in 63–80% of patients with epidermal or mixed type of melasma after 6 months. Since treatment of melasma with azelaic acid requires several months, a combination of azelaic acid with other drugs deserves consideration [13].

Medium-depth chemical peeling has been used alone in the treatment of melasma; however, sometimes this treatment may result in worsening of the hyperpigmented lesion. A combined treatment with 35% trichloracetic acid peel followed by 4% hydroquinone acetate cream and 0.05% tretinoin cream was reported to be effective for epidermal and mixed-type melasma in fair-skinned women. The response of melasma to chemical peeling is, however, unpredictable, and may be aggravated as a result of postinflammatory hyperpigmentation. In general, chemical peeling should not be used in dark-skinned individuals [13].

The treatment of melasma with various types of lasers has been tried, but without significant success. The use of a 510 nm dye laser, resulted in failure and sometimes even in hyperpigmentation. Use of Q-switched ruby lasers has good results initially, but a quick recurrence occurs when the treatment is stopped [13]. The copper vapor laser and the argon laser also failed to show improvement in patients with melasma [10]. The use of lasers during pregnancy has not been studied [25].

In conclusion, the important aspect of treatment is stressing the natural course of hyper-melanosis, since improvement is expected postpartum. Reassuring is thus a major contributor to treatment.

Summary

> Hyperpigmentation during pregnancy is a very common condition, affecting mainly the areolae, genital skin, and linea alba. This condition usually regresses after parturition.
> Melasma is hyperpigmentation of the face, which occurs in 45–75% of pregnant women. Melasma may also be seen with oral contraceptive pills. It may occur in three clinical patterns – centrofacial, malar, and mandibular – and histologically in two types – epidermal and dermal. UV light radiation plays a major etiologic role.
> Hyperpigmentation in pregnancy has been attributed to increased output of some combination of placental, pituitary, and ovarian hormones – namely, melanocyte-simulating hormone, estrogen, progesterone, and bioactive sphingolipids derived from the placenta.
> Treatment of pigmentary alterations during pregnancy consists mainly of reassurance, prevention of sun exposure, and the use of sunscreens.

References

1. Barankin B, Silver SG, Carruthers A (2002) The skin in pregnancy. J Cutan Med Surg 6:236–240
2. Beischer NA, Wein P (1996) Linea alba pigmentation and umbilical deviation in nulliparous pregnancy: the ligamentum teres sign. Obstet Gynecol 87:254–256
3. Clark D, Thody AJ, Shuster S et al (1978) Immunoreactive alpha-MSH in human plasma in pregnancy. Nature 273:163–164
4. Dahlberg BC (1961) Melanocyte stimulating substances in the urine of pregnant women. Acta Endocrinol Suppl (Copenh) 38(Suppl 60):1–51
5. Elling SV, Powell FC (1997) Physiological changes in the skin during pregnancy. Clin Dermatol 15:35–43
6. Ellis DL, Wheeland RG (1986) Increased nevus estrogen and progesterone ligand binding related to oral contraceptives or pregnancy. J Am Acad Dermatol 14:25–31
7. Errickson CV, Matus NR (1994) Skin disorders of pregnancy. Am Fam Physician 49:605–610
8. Eudy SF, Baker GF (1990) Dermatopathology for the obstetrician. Clin Obstet Gynecol 33:728–737
9. Fryer JM, Werth VP (1992) Pregnancy-associated hyperpigmentation: longitudinal melanonychia. J Am Acad Dermatol 26:493–494
10. Grimes PE (1995) Melasma. Etiologic and therapeutic considerations. Arch Dermatol 131:1453–1457
11. Hellreich P (1974) The skin changes of pregnancy. Cutis 13:82–86
12. James WD, Meltzer MS, Guill MA et al (1984) Pigmentary demarcation lines associated with pregnancy. J Am Acad Dermatol 11:438–440
13. Katsambas A, Antoniou C (1995) Melasma. Classification and treatment. J Eur Acad Dermatol Venereol 4:217
14. Kligman AM, Willis I (1975) A new formula for depigmenting human skin. Arch Dermatol 111:40–48
15. Kumari R, Laxmisha C, Thappa DM (2006) Pigmentary demarcation lines associated with pregnancy. J Cosmet Dermatol 5:169–170
16. Kumari R, Jaisankar TJ, Thappa DM (2007) A clinical study of skin changes in pregnancy. Indian J Dermatol Venereol Leprol 73:141
17. Mallick S, Singh SK, Sarkar C et al (2005) Human placental lipid induces melanogenesis by increasing the expression of tyrosinase and its related proteins in vitro. Pigment Cell Res 18:25–33
18. Martin AG, Leal-Khouri S (1992) Physiologic skin changes associated with pregnancy. Int J Dermatol 31:375–378
19. McGuinness B (1963) Melanocyte-stimulating hormone. A clinical and laboratory study. Ann N Y Acad Sci 100:640–657
20. McKenzie AW (1971) Skin disorders in pregnancy. Practitioner 206:773–780
21. Muallem MM, Rubeiz NG (2006) Physiological and biological skin changes in pregnancy. Clin Dermatol 24:80–83
22. Murray JC (1990) Pregnancy and the skin. Dermatol Clin 8:327–334
23. Muzaffar F, Hussain I, Haroon TS (1998) Physiologic skin changes during pregnancy: a study of 140 cases. Int J Dermatol 37:429–431
24. Newcomer VD, Lindberg MC, Sternberg TH (1961) A melanosis of the face ("chloasma"). Arch Dermatol 83:284–299
25. Nussbaum R, Benedetto AV (2006) Cosmetic aspects of pregnancy. Clin Dermatol 24:133–141

26. Ozawa H, Rokugo M, Aoyama H (1993) Pigmentary demarcation lines of pregnancy with erythema. Dermatology 187:134–136

27. Parmley T, O'Brien TJ (1990) Skin changes during pregnancy. Clin Obstet Gynecol 33: 713–717

28. Perez M, Sanchez JL, Aguilo F (1983) Endocrinologic profile of patients with idiopathic melasma. J Invest Dermatol 81:543–545

29. Raj S, Khopkar U, Kapasi A et al (1992) Skin in pregnancy. Indian Dermatol Venereol Leprol 58:84–88

30. Ranson M, Posen S, Mason RS (1988) Human melanocytes as a target tissue for hormones: in vitro studies with 1 alpha-25, dihydroxyvitamin D3, alpha-melanocyte stimulating hormone, and beta-estradiol. J Invest Dermatol 91:593–598

31. Rubin AI, Laborde SV, Stiller MJ (2001) Acquired dermal melanocytosis: appearance during pregnancy. J Am Acad Dermatol 45:609–613

32. Sanchez NP, Pathak MA, Sato S et al (1981) Melasma: a clinical, light microscopic, ultrastructural, and immunofluorescence study. J Am Acad Dermatol 4:698–710

33. Shizume K, Lerner AB (1954) Determination of melanocyte-stimulating hormone in urine and blood. J Clin Endocrinol Metab 14:1491–1510

34. Snell RS, Bischitz PG (1960) The effect of large doses of estrogen and estrogen and progesterone on melanin pigmentation. J Invest Dermatol 35:73–82

35. Szabo G (1954) The number of melanocytes in human epidermis. Br Med J 1:1016–1017

36. Thody AJ, Plummer NA, Burton JL et al (1974) Plasma beta-melanocyte-stimulating hormone levels in pregnancy. J Obstet Gynaecol Br Commonw 81:875–877

37. Vazquez M, Ibanez MI, Sanchez JL (1986) Pigmentary demarcation lines during pregnancy. Cutis 38:263–266

38. Wade TR, Wade SL, Jones HE (1978) Skin changes and diseases associated with pregnancy. Obstet Gynecol 52:233–242

39. Winton GB, Lewis CW (1982) Dermatoses of pregnancy. J Am Acad Dermatol 6:977–998

40. Wong RC, Ellis CN (1984) Physiologic skin changes in pregnancy. J Am Acad Dermatol 10:929–940

41. Wong RC, Ellis CN (1989) Physiologic skin changes in pregnancy. Semin Dermatol 8:7–11

3.1
Hair

3.1.1
Hirsutism

Hirsutism is defined as excessive hair growth in both a normal and an abnormal distribution [13]. Most pregnant women develop some degree of hirsutism, which is usually most pronounced on the face (upper lip, chin, and cheeks). The arms, legs, and back can also be involved (Figs. 3.1, 3.2) [22, 23]. In addition, suprapubic midline hair growth with a male-pattern distribution may also be increased during pregnancy [5, 23]. Acne may be an accompanying feature of hirsutism [23].

Hirsutism generally starts early in pregnancy, and is usually more pronounced in women with preexisting abundant body hair or very dark hair or in women with a preexisting tendency toward a male pattern of hair distribution [4, 23]. Within 6 months postpartum and even before delivery, most of the excess fine lanugo hairs disappear, but coarse and bristly hair usually remains. Recurrence with subsequent pregnancies is common [23].

Scalp hair becomes fuller during pregnancy, which correlates with an increase in the hair mean shaft diameter when compared with the nonpregnant state. This increase was found to start at the beginning of pregnancy [12, 13].

The hair cycle consists of three phases: anagen, catagen, and telogen. The anagen phase is the growth phase of hair, includes 85% of scalp hair, and lasts 3 years. The catagen (transition) phase lasts 2–3 weeks and evolves into the telogen (rest) phase, which lasts 3 months until the hair eventually sheds [1]. Each follicle has its own rhythm, uninfluenced by its attaching follicle and usually out of phase with the rhythms of its neighbors [9].

Lynfield [9] observed the hair roots of 26 women during and after normal pregnancies. The mean percentage of anagen hairs in the first trimester was 85%, which was similar to that of nonpregnant controls. By the second trimester, the percentage increased to 95%, and this proportion was maintained through the first week postpartum. This may parallel

A. Ingber, *Obstetric Dermatology*,
DOI: 10.1007/978-3-540-88399-9, © Springer-Verlag Berlin Heidelberg 2009

3

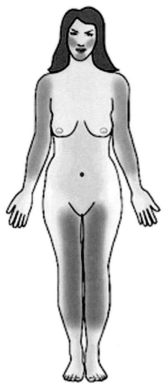
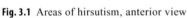
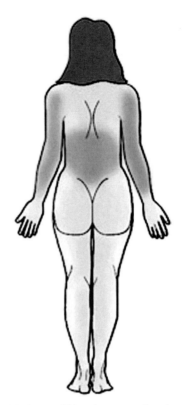

Fig. 3.1 Areas of hirsutism, anterior view   **Fig. 3.2** Areas of hirsutism, posterior view

the vigor of hair growth claimed by many pregnant women. This change was suggested to be as a result of slowed conversion of hair from anagen hair to telogen hair. An alternative possibility was that pregnancy is associated with a more rapid shedding of telogen hairs. It is interesting to note that, in an earlier study of seven women conducted by Trotter [19], no variations in rate of hair growth were observed in the pubic, perianal, and lumbar regions that could be attributed to the pregnancy.

Two cases of general hypertrichosis during pregnancy, which disappeared postpartum, were described by Stoddard [17]. In those cases the hair growth was especially prominent on the face. These changes were attributed to an excess of corticosteroids, analogous to the hirsutism of Cushing's syndrome. It was later suggested [9] that in those cases the cycle of facial and body hair is altered in the same way as that of scalp hair, based on the same hormonal changes.

The observed alterations of the hair cycle by pregnancy were explained by changed endocrine assemblage [9]. Increased adrenocorticotrophic hormone and adrenocorticosteroid secretion, as well as augmented ovarian androgen secretion, may account for the increase in anagen hairs and subsequent hirsutism [23].

In animal experiments, hormonal influences on the hair cycle have been clearly demonstrated. Among the observed effects, the most significant observation has been that estrogens prolong the anagen phase once a cycle has begun [9]. There are abundant β-type estrogen receptors (the major steroid receptor expressed in human skin) expressed within the hair follicle. This expression is localized to nuclei of outer root sheath, epithelial matrix, and dermal papilla cells. It is likely that higher levels of estrogen binding to these receptors induce changes that keep follicles in the anagen phase of the hair growth cycle [13, 18].

Severe abnormalities of hair growth and virilization are occasionally seen in association with fetal malformation and stillbirth, but the mechanism for these is still not completely understood [11]. It was suggested that patients with marked hirsutism can be studied closely for virilizing tumors [22], and thus tumors of the ovary, luteomas, lutein cysts, or polycystic ovary disease should be excluded [23].

Treatment consists of education, reassurance, and cosmetic treatment of unwanted hair postpartum. There are plenty permanent and nonpermanent options for treating hirsutism. These include shaving, waxing, electrolysis, and laser epilation. Lasers have become very popular and effective in recent years. Treatment is usually postponed until after parturition because the effects of lasers during pregnancy have not been definitively determined [13]. Most physicians recommend waiting 6 months before starting treatment [1, 23, 24].

3.1.2 Telogen Effluvium

Shortly after parturition, Lynfield [9] found a decrease in the percentage of anagen follicles to 76%, probably as a result of accelerated conversion from anagen hair to telogen hair. This hair loss has been termed "telogen effluvium." Telogen effluvium is a nonspecific pattern of hair loss brought on by a variety of stimuli, usually stress [21]. It is classified together with postinfectious, postoperative, and posttraumatic hair loss. These alopecias have in common their diffuseness and their good prognosis [9]. Another constant feature of this phenomenon is a latent period between the stress and the hair-shedding process [21]. Histologically, there are normal follicles in telogen hair without dysplastic changes [21]. This shedding of hair actually represents reactivation of the hair follicle and new growth [5].

This shedding generally lasts 1–5 months, but may not cease until 15 months postpartum [8]. Sabouraud [15] described that hair loss postpartum begins suddenly 70–75 days after childbirth, and lasts 6 weeks. According to Lynfield [9], the time of onset and duration of postpartum hair loss was variable. It began almost immediately after delivery in two women, 1 month postpartum in one, and 4 months postpartum in another. This condition lasted up to 5 months. In a study of 35 postpartum women with hair loss [7], shedding began 2–4 months after parturition, and it continued for 2–5 months, but occasionally considerably longer. In a study of 98 patients, Schiff and Kern [16] reported that in almost 90% of cases hair loss began between 8 and 16 weeks postpartum. In this study two thirds of patients returned to normal in 4–6 months. The anterior scalp was involved in 59.1% of cases, in 20.4% of cases it was diffuse over the entire scalp, and in 11.2% of cases the frontal regions alone were involved [16]. A longer interval of telogen effluvium could be due to individually longer catagen–telogen times or possibly persistent partial cyclic synchrony [6].

Although complete hair regrowth usually occurs, the hair may not be as abundant as it was prior to pregnancy [23], and women often complain that the density is not the same as that before pregnancy [13]. Patients sometimes complain of apparent postpartum changes in

3

hair color, texture, and curliness. It is also possible that there might be temporary or even permanent changes in the duration of the anagen phase that could simultaneously result in slight but persistent increased hair loss accompanied by a decrease in achievable hair length [6].

The cause of postpartum telogen effluvium may involve multiple factors, including the stress of delivery (fever, surgical stress, emotional stress, and blood loss) and changes in endocrine balance [23]. Behrman [2] postulated that postpartum alopecia may be the result of an estrogen deficiency state, resulting from an inhibiting effect on the gonadotrophic activities of the anterior pituitary gland by the high steroid levels occurring during pregnancy.

Postpartum telogen effluvium is often not recognized by the family physician. This may be accompanied by skepticism about the presence of hair loss and suspicion of a phobic state [11]. It is helpful to remember that 25% of the scalp hair must be lost before clearly identifiable thinning occurs. The hair loss in this condition may be severe, but complete and spontaneous regrowth is the rule [11]. This event is more or less reproducible in succeeding pregnancies, although this is not certain [6].

Since this condition has an excellent prognosis, reassurance should be the most important therapeutic modality. Since hair loss is an extremely worrisome experience to women, the physician should notify the patient with postpartum alopecia that what she is experiencing is a normal physiologic response to hormonal alterations [16]. It should be stressed, however, that confidently predicting hair growth will always return to the normal prepregnancy state is not recommended [6]. In those cases where a seborrheic component appears to be present, antiseborrheic therapy is helpful in preventing hair loss that may be on that basis [16].

3.1.3
Male-Pattern Baldness and Hypotrichosis

Rarely, a mild degree of frontoparietal recession characteristic of male-pattern alopecia is seen toward the end of pregnancy, usually in women with a tendency toward androgenetic alopecia. In addition, diffuse thinning of the hair can occur late in pregnancy. Again, spontaneous recovery occurs [11, 14, 20]; however, some investigators disagree, and claim that complete regrowth of hair is not to be expected [21].

The causes of male-pattern baldness and hypotrichosis are unknown, but inhibition of gonadotrophic activity secondary to high steroid levels may play an important role [10].

3.2
Nails

Nail changes are uncommon in pregnancy; when they do occur, they usually appear as early as the sixth week and consist of increased brittleness and softening, distal onycholysis (separation of the nail plate from the nail bed, similar to that seen occasionally in thyrotoxicosis), and subungual keratosis [3, 5, 10, 22, 23]. None of these changes are unique to pregnancy [5]. Beau's lines are transverse grooves in the nails and are caused by temporary impairment of nail plate formation by the nail matrix [5]. These lines may develop after delivery [10]. The nail changes usually regress in 6 months to 1 year postpartum [10]. Nail growth is generally increased during pregnancy and slows postpartum [3].

The pathogenesis of these changes is not known, and their relationship to pregnancy is unclear; therefore, other cases should be eliminated when these changes are observed [22]. When brittleness and distal onycholysis are observed, other causes of the onychodystrophy such as psoriasis, lichen planus, or onychomycosis should be excluded [5]. Nail changes in pregnancy are usually benign and do not require treatment other than reassurance and promotion of good nail care [1, 20]. An attempt should be made to avoid external sensitizers (nail polish, nail removers) and infections [23]. The nails should be kept short if they are brittle or prone to onycholysis [23].

Summary

> Most pregnant women develop hirsutism, most marked on the face, limbs, and back. This condition regresses in 6 months, but usually coarse hairs remain. During pregnancy, there is a higher percentage of follicles in the anagen phase.

> Telogen effluvium is a condition of hair shedding which starts 1–5 months postpartum and may last up to 2 years. Complete hair regrowth usually occurs.

> Rarely, male-pattern alopecia is seen during the end of pregnancy, usually in women with a tendency toward androgenetic alopecia. Spontaneous recovery usually occurs.

> Nail changes are uncommon in pregnancy, and may include brittleness, onycholysis, and subungual keratosis. Other diseases should be eliminated when nail changes are observed.

References

1. Barankin B, Silver SG, Carruthers A (2002) The skin in pregnancy. J Cutan Med Surg 6:236–240
2. Behrman H (1952) The scalp in health and disease. Mosby, St Louis
3. Elling SV, Powell FC (1997) Physiological changes in the skin during pregnancy. Clin Dermatol 15:35–43
4. Errickson CV, Matus NR (1994) Skin disorders of pregnancy. Am Fam Physician 49:605–610
5. Eudy SF, Baker GF (1990) Dermatopathology for the obstetrician. Clin Obstet Gynecol 33:728–737
6. Headington JT (1993) Telogen effluvium. New concepts and review. Arch Dermatol 129:356–363
7. Kligman A (1961) Pathologic dynamics of human hair loss. 1- Telogen effluvium. Arch Dermatol 83:175–198
8. Kroumpouzos G, Cohen LM (2001) Dermatoses of pregnancy. J Am Acad Dermatol 45:1–19; quiz 19–22
9. Lynfield YL (1960) Effect of pregnancy on the human hair cycle. J Invest Dermatol 35:323–327
10. Martin AG, Leal-Khouri S (1992) Physiologic skin changes associated with pregnancy. Int J Dermatol 31:375–378
11. McKenzie AW (1971) Skin disorders in pregnancy. Practitioner 206:773–780

12. Nissimov J, Elchalal U (2003) Scalp hair diameter increases during pregnancy. Clin Exp Dermatol 28:525–530
13. Nussbaum R, Benedetto AV (2006) Cosmetic aspects of pregnancy. Clin Dermatol 24:133–141
14. Parmley T, O'Brien TJ (1990) Skin changes during pregnancy. Clin Obstet Gynecol 33:713–717
15. Sabouraud R (1936) Alopecias. Masson et Cie, Paris
16. Schiff BL, Kern AB (1963) Study of postpartum alopecia. Arch Dermatol 87:609–611
17. Stoddard F (1945) Hirsutism in pregnancy. Am J Obstet Gynecol 49:417–422
18. Thornton MJ, Taylor AH, Mulligan K et al (2003) Oestrogen receptor beta is the predominant oestrogen receptor in human scalp skin. Exp Dermatol 12:181–190
19. Trotter M (1935) The activity of hair follicles with reference to pregnancy. Surg Gynecol Obstet 60:1092–1096
20. Tunzi M, Gray GR (2007) Common skin conditions during pregnancy. Am Fam Physician 75:211–218
21. Wade TR, Wade SL, Jones HE (1978) Skin changes and diseases associated with pregnancy. Obstet Gynecol 52:233–242
22. Winton GB, Lewis CW (1982) Dermatoses of pregnancy. J Am Acad Dermatol 6:977–998
23. Wong RC, Ellis CN (1984) Physiologic skin changes in pregnancy. J Am Acad Dermatol 10:929–940
24. Wong RC, Ellis CN (1989) Physiologic skin changes in pregnancy. Semin Dermatol 8:7–11

Connective Tissue Physiologic Changes During Pregnancy

4

4.1
Striae Distensae
(Linea Striae, Linea Gravidarum, Linea Alba, Striae Gravidarum)

These linear stretch marks are a prominent feature of most pregnancies, and they develop in 90% of white pregnant women [34, 37]. They are uncommon in black and Asian women, and appear to have a familial tendency [34, 37]. They are not associated only with pregnancy, and can be seen to a lesser degree in 35% of adolescents, appearing in girls 2.5 times more frequently than in boys [31].

These stretch marks are irregular in shape, purple–red–violaceous, wrinkled, slightly depressed streaks which finally become white and usually occur at about the sixth to the seventh month of pregnancy. They tend to occur in areas of maximum stretch, and develop initially opposite to the skin tension lines on the abdomen [18, 34, 37]. They often spread to involve the breasts, lower portion of the back, buttocks, thighs, upper arms, axillae, and inguinal areas (Figs. 4.1–4.4) [11, 37], and are sometimes accompanied by pruritus [19]. It was speculated that physical factors dictate their localization and direction, since they were found to appear on the expanding girth of the abdomen in pregnancy and after repeated trauma in adolescents [13, 18, 28]. There is, however, no correlation between the enlargement of body size during pregnancy and the intensity of striation [34].

The cause of striae is still unclear, and, according to many investigators, is a combination of distension and adrenocortical activity [6, 24, 34, 37], in addition to a genetic predisposition [16]. Several studies support the opinion that they are probably influenced more by increased adrenocortical activity rather than by increased abdominal circumference [37], and, indeed, Poidevin [24] found a relationship with increased adrenocortical activity, but no correlation with increased abdominal girth. Studies that support the role of corticosteroids in striae development are numerous. Epstein et al. [9] reported the development of atrophic inguinal striae in five men, ages 16–39, after the prolonged use of a topical steroid cream for intertrigo. Chernosky and Knox [5] reported the development of atrophic atriae in two young girls treated with occlusive corticosteroid dressings at the

A. Ingber, *Obstetric Dermatology*,
DOI: 10.1007/978-3-540-88399-9, © Springer-Verlag Berlin Heidelberg 2009

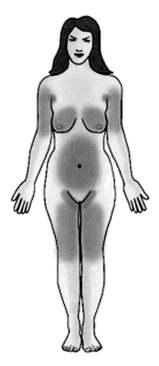

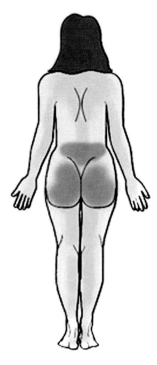

Fig. 4.1 Areas of involvement of striae distensae, anterior view

Fig. 4.2 Areas of involvement of striae distensae, posterior view

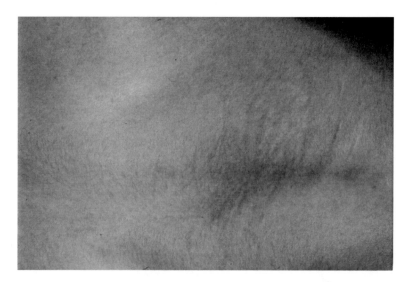

Fig. 4.3 Striae distensae. Low back of a pregnant women. Note pigmentation on the same site

Fig. 4.4 Striae distensae. The same woman as in Fig. 4.3. Close view of the striae and of the pigmentation

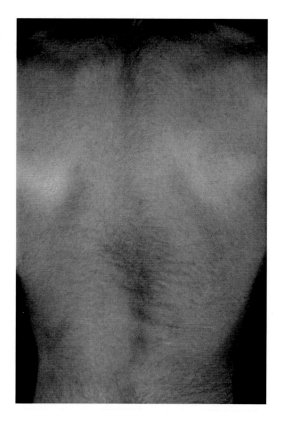

sites of occlusion. A comparison between obese persons with and without striae found increased excretion of corticosteroids in the ones with striae [30]. These studies are further supported by reports of striae development in Cushing's syndrome and in patients treated with systemic corticosteroids [18].

Corticosteroids appear to generate weakening and rupture of dermal elastic fibers, which are seen histologically as twisted strands at the periphery of the lesions, and are absent in the center of the streaks. Collagen fibers stain weakly and are disposed discreetly rather than in interwoven bundles in the dermis [18].

Liu [16] proposed in 1974 that a series of events which happen during pregnancy lead to the formation of stretch marks. The first stage is "priming" of the skin by relaxin, a hormone which increases during pregnancy, and estrogen. These hormones cause an increase in the production of collagen and sulfate-free mucopolysaccharides. The "primed" connective tissue is then subjected to stretching. Liu also proposed that the increase in relaxin, estrogen, and corticosteroid levels during pregnancy leads to the formation of sulfate-free mucopolysaccharides. Water absorption by these mucopolysaccharides relaxes the interfibrous cohesive forces, leading to a cleavage or fraying of the collagen fibers, which then easily separate. He proposed that without priming of the dermis, no striae would form when the skin is stretched. However, Shuster [29] believed that stretch with intradermal tears of collagen is the sole factor in striae gravidarum, without the need for the "priming" stage.

Later, Watson et al. [35] suggested that changes in the skin elements necessary for tensile strength and elasticity, namely, fibrillin, elastin, and collagen, are suspected in the development of striae gravidarum. Their study was conducted on skin biopsies from early erythematous striae and adjacent normal skin in pregnant women. By using electron microscopy, light microscopy, and immunohistochemistry, they found differences that included looser dermal matrix, increased levels of glycosaminoglycans, reduced levels of fibrillin and elastic fibers, and alterations in the orientation of elastin and fibrillin in the dermis. These researchers raised the question of whether the constant stretch of pregnancy might lead to remodeling of the dermis, but this question remains unanswered [22].

The fact that striae may also be observed in patients with obesity, diabetes, Cushing's syndrome, Marfan's syndrome, steroid therapy, tuberculosis, and rapid weight increase or decrease implies that several different pathways may lead to the same clinical pictures [7,21]. It should be noted that the cutaneous changes of pruritic urticarial papules and plaques of pregnancy, a condition that typically affects primigravidas (see Chap. 18), is typically localized to abdominal striae in its onset. This suggests that striae damage of the skin leads to a possible exposure of antigenic foci, with secondary inflammatory reactions [7, 25].

There seems to be a significant association between the incidence of striae and heavier babies as well as heavier or obese mothers [6]. A recent report by Thomas and Liston [32] found that striae gravidarum were associated with higher body mass index as well as baby weight, supporting this previous report. In addition, they reported that advancing age was inversely proportional to the development of striae. It was also believed that striae are associated with increased abdominal wall thickness [6].

A large study conducted lately reported that 50% of patients with striae gravidarum had mothers with striae gravidarum [4]. However, the strongest association was made between striae gravidarum and the presence of breast and thigh striae. Eighty-one percent of women with striae gravidarum had preexisting striae on the breasts and thighs. In contrast, only 31% of women without striae gravidarum had striae in these locations. In contrast to previous reports, this study did not find a correlation between body mass index or degree of weight gain and striae gravidarum development. The authors noted, however, that since very few women in the study were obese these results may be biased. Taken as a whole, genetics as well as possible variations in the ultrastructural composition of the dermis seem to play a major role in the development of striae gravidarum [4, 22].

Striae associated with pregnancy usually gradually fade after parturition to pale atrophic lines, but they do not fade completely [13, 34, 36].

Striae often comprise a cosmetic problem, but, unfortunately, therapy remains unsatisfactory [7, 19]. Optional therapies include preventive measures during pregnancy and postpartum therapy. In prevention, there is controversy as to the effectiveness of olive oil and massage [6, 24]. Davey [6] found that abdominal striae were significantly less common when the skin had been massaged with oil; however, Poidevin [24] reported that not only nightly rubbing of olive oil fails as a prophylactic, but it actually appeared to predispose to the development of striae. In addition, it should be emphasized that the application of vitamin E and aloe oil, in addition to not being proven to work, may also be associated with a contact dermatitis reaction [1]. Other suggested preventive topical measures, which are not always beneficial, include the application of creams containing α-tocopherol, collagen–elastin hydrolysates, and *Centella asiatica* extract, an East Asian medicinal plant containing pentacyclic triterpene derivatives [3, 38]. Another suggested treatment contains tocopherol, essential fatty acids, panthenol, hyaluronic acid, elastin, and menthol [33]. Neither of these products is widely available, and the safety of using *Centella asiatica* during pregnancy and the components responsible for their effectiveness has not been fully elucidated [10]. One report describes personal successful experience in preventing striae gravidarum in all pregnant patients with a combination of zinc, ascorbic acid, pyridoxal, and flaxseed oil; however, no large study was conducted to test this observation [15].

Tretinoin has been reported to be of limited effectiveness in postpartum treatment of striae distensae [8]. An open-label study with 0.1% tretinoin cream showed a decrease in the severity of striae gravidarum after 3 months of application [27]. However, a double-blind placebo-controlled trial of 0.025% tretinoin cream applied for 7 months to striae gravidarum failed to demonstrate significant improvements over the placebo [26]. Oral tretinoin therapy was also suggested as a potential postpartum therapy [33]. Excimer (308 nm) and pulsed dye (585 nm) lasers have shown limited effects in the treatment of striae [12, 14, 17, 20]. Surgical excision of striae with abdominoplasty has favorable results when there is accompanying redundant abdominal skin [22].

It is important to reassure the pregnant woman that with time the discoloration will probably become less noticeable, but she also should be told that the stretch marks will persist [34].

4.2
Molluscum Fibrosum Gravidarum

These lesions, also known as acrochordons, were first reported by Brickner [2] in 1906. The lesions he described are small, up to 5 mm in size, flesh-colored or slightly hyperpigmented, and polypoid. They are usually located in the axillae, the groin, inframammary areas, on the side of the neck, on the face, on the chest, and occasionally on the feet [7, 23]. They are identical to skin tags as seen clinically in normal or obese individuals [7]. Histologically, they reveal papules with hyperkeratosis, papillomatosis, and acanthosis, similar to normal skin tags [1]. The dermis has loose collagen and a paucity of adnexal structures [1]. Their onset is during the fourth to sixth months of pregnancy and they usually disappear after parturition. In some patients they sometimes persist and undergo continued increase in size during following pregnancies. Although the cause of these lesions is unclear, many authors believe that they are probably due to the hormonal growth factor element of the endocrine environment of pregnancy [7, 34]. They have no malignant potential [23], and unlike warts they are not of viral origin and therefore are not infective [7]. Treatment with liquid nitrogen, electrocautery, or simple shave excision under local anesthetic is effective for persistent lesions [7].

4

Summary

› Striae distensae appear in 90% of pregnant women during the sixth to seventh months as purple streaks.
› Their cause is still unknown, but is probably a combination of distension and adrenocortical activity.
› They usually gradually fade after parturition to pale atrophic lines, but they do not fade completely.
› Preventive measures by different topical therapies are controversial. Optional postpartum treatments include tretinoin, laser therapy, and surgical excision.
› Molluscum fibrosum gravidarum are small lesions identical to skin tags. They usually disappear after delivery, but in some women they may persist.

References

1. Barankin B, Silver SG, Carruthers A (2002) The skin in pregnancy. J Cutan Med Surg 6:236–240
2. Brickner S (1906) Fibroma molluscum gravidarum: a new clinical entity. Am J Obstet Gynecol 53:191–198
3. Brinkhaus B, Lindner M, Schuppan D et al (2000) Chemical, pharmacological and clinical profile of the East Asian medical plant Centella asiatica. Phytomedicine 7:427–448
4. Chang AL, Agredano YZ, Kimball AB (2004) Risk factors associated with striae gravidarum. J Am Acad Dermatol 51:881–885
5. Chernosky ME, Knox JM (1964) Atrophic striae after occlusive corticosteroid therapy. Arch Dermatol 90:15–19
6. Davey CM (1972) Factors associated with the occurrence of striae gravidarum. J Obstet Gynaecol Br Commonw 79:1113–1114
7. Elling SV, Powell FC (1997) Physiological changes in the skin during pregnancy. Clin Dermatol 15:35–43
8. Elson ML (1990) Treatment of striae distensae with topical tretinoin. J Dermatol Surg Oncol 16:267–270
9. Epstein N, Epstein W, Epstein J (1963) Atopic striae in patients with inguinal intertrigo. Arch Dermatol 87:450
10. Ernst E (2002) Herbal medicinal products during pregnancy: are they safe? BJOG 109:227–235
11. Eudy SF, Baker GF (1990) Dermatopathology for the obstetrician. Clin Obstet Gynecol 33:728–737
12. Goldberg DJ, Sarradet D, Hussain M (2003) 308-nm excimer laser treatment of mature hypopigmented striae. Dermatol Surg 29:596–598; discussion 598–599
13. Hellreich P (1974) The skin changes of pregnancy. Cutis 13:82–86
14. Jimenez GP, Flores F, Berman B et al (2003) Treatment of striae rubra and striae alba with the 585-nm pulsed-dye laser. Dermatol Surg 29:362–365
15. Levin WM (1995) Striae gravidarum: folklore and fact. Arch Fam Med 4:98.
16. Liu DT (1974) Letter: striae gravidarum. Lancet 1:625
17. McDaniel DH (2002) Laser therapy of stretch marks. Dermatol Clin 20:67–76, viii

18. McKenzie AW (1971) Skin disorders in pregnancy. Practitioner 206:773–780
19. Muallem MM, Rubeiz NG (2006) Physiological and biological skin changes in pregnancy. Clin Dermatol 24:80–83
20. Nehal KS, Lichtenstein DA, Kamino H et al (1999) Treatment of mature striae with the pulsed dye laser. J Cutan Laser Ther 1:41–44
21. Nigam PK (1989) Striae cutis distensae. Int J Dermatol 28:426–428
22. Nussbaum R, Benedetto AV (2006) Cosmetic aspects of pregnancy. Clin Dermatol 24:133–141
23. Parmley T, O'Brien TJ (1990) Skin changes during pregnancy. Clin Obstet Gynecol 33:713–717
24. Poidevin LO (1959) Striae gravidarum. Their relation to adrenal cortical hyperfunction. Lancet 2:436–439
25. Powell F, Dervan P, Wayte J, O'Loughlin S (1996) Pruritic urticarial papules and plaques of pregnancy (PUPPP): a clinicopathological review of 35 patients. J Eur Acad Dermatol Venereol 6:105–111
26. Pribanich S, Simpson FG, Held B et al (1994) Low-dose tretinoin does not improve striae distensae: a double-blind, placebo-controlled study. Cutis 54:121–124
27. Rangel O, Arias I, Garcia E et al (2001) Topical tretinoin 0.1% for pregnancy-related abdominal striae: an open-label, multicenter, prospective study. Adv Ther 18:181–186
28. Shelley WB, Cohen W (1964) Stria migrans. Arch Dermatol 90:193–194
29. Shuster S (1979) The cause of striae distensae. Acta Derm Venereol Suppl (Stockh) 59:161–169
30. Simkin B, Arce R (1962) Steroid excretion in obese patients with colored abdominal striae. N Engl J Med 266:1031–1035
31. Sisson WR (1954) Colored striae in adolescent children. J Pediatr 45:520–530
32. Thomas RG, Liston WA (2004) Clinical associations of striae gravidarum. J Obstet Gynaecol 24:270–271
33. Tunzi M, Gray GR (2007) Common skin conditions during pregnancy. Am Fam Physician 75:211–218
34. Wade TR, Wade SL, Jones HE (1978) Skin changes and diseases associated with pregnancy. Obstet Gynecol 52:233–242
35. Watson RE, Parry EJ, Humphries JD et al (1998) Fibrillin microfibrils are reduced in skin exhibiting striae distensae. Br J Dermatol 138:931–937
36. Winton GB, Lewis CW (1982) Dermatoses of pregnancy. J Am Acad Dermatol 6:977–998
37. Wong RC, Ellis CN (1984) Physiologic skin changes in pregnancy. J Am Acad Dermatol 10:929–940
38. Young GL, Jewell D (2000) Creams for preventing stretch marks in pregnancy. Cochrane Database Syst Rev CD000066. doi:10.1002/14651858.CD000066

Physiologic Vascular Changes During Pregnancy

5

Vascular changes are frequent during pregnancy, and occur to a variable extent in women. The changes include distension, instability, and proliferation of vessels [38]. The main clinical results of these abnormalities are spider angiomata (nevi aranei) and palmar erythema [35]. Other commonly seen abnormalities are flushing of the skin and temporary edema of the face, hands, and feet [24]. Most rare are small hemangiomas of subcutaneous cavernous type which disappear shortly after delivery [24].

Some of the vascular changes are used as diagnostic features of pregnancy. Erythema of the vestibule and vagina, called the Jacquemier–Chadwick sign, results from distension of their vasculature, and occurs early in gestation [19, 38]. The bluish discoloration of the cervix, known as the Goodell sign, is also a result of increased vascularity, this time of the cervix [7].

The most remarkable vascular change is simply general vascular increase throughout the dermis. This can lead to significant blood loss encountered by a simple incision in the skin of a pregnant woman [7], and this tendency may jeopardize the course of a cesarean section [7].

5.1
Vascular Spiders (Spider Angiomas, Arterial Spiders, Nevi Aranei, Spider Nevi)

Spider nevi are seen in 10–15% of normal white, nonpregnant women. During pregnancy their number markedly increases, and they are found in about 70% of whites and 10–15% of blacks [13, 24, 40]. The prevalence of vascular spiders in pregnant women reported by Bean [3] in a large series was 67% among whites and 11.3% among blacks by the third trimester. Esteve et al. [9] reported that 32 out of 60 pregnant women developed vascular spiders, most of them appearing on the upper part of the body, and only one vascular spider was seen on the leg. In a study of 140 pregnant women from Lahore, Pakistan, by Muzaffar et al. [27], a very low incidence of spider nevi, 1.4%, was reported. This difference was credited in part to the dark complexion of the women, making the nevi less perceptible.

A. Ingber, *Obstetric Dermatology*, DOI: 10.1007/978-3-540-88399-9, © Springer-Verlag Berlin Heidelberg 2009

5

Spider nevi usually appear between the second and fifth months of pregnancy [13]. The study by Bean et al. [4] found that 14% of white women had spider angiomata by the second month of pregnancy, but African-American women developed them only after the fourth month of pregnancy. There is a tendency for them to increase in size and number until parturition [35]. Clinically, spider nevi appear as small, flat, or slightly raised lesions with a central, faintly pulsating, red punctum associated with small, radiating, telangiectatic vessels, and surrounding erythema, usually extending several millimeters beyond the visible vessels [35, 39]. The temperature of the skin overlying the spider nevi is warmer than that of the neighboring skin [28]. Pressure on the central point will produce blanching [29].

Spider nevi occur mostly in areas of skin drained by the superior vena cava, the neck, throat, face (particularly around the eyes), upper chest, arms, and hands (in that order) (Figs. 5.1, 5.2) and consist of a central artery containing muscle and glomus cells in its thick wall, arising from the subcutaneous arterial plexus [13, 24, 38, 39]. In the subepidermal zone the artery dilates into a thin-walled ampulla giving off delicate arterial branches which merge into the capillary bed [24]. Following delivery, their size and number gradu-

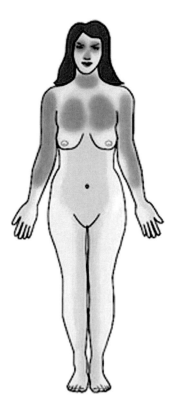

Fig. 5.1 Areas of involvement of spider nevi

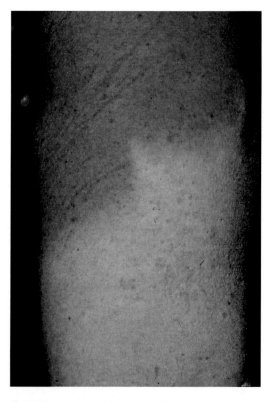

Fig. 5.2 Numerous spider nevi in a pregnant woman

ally decrease [35]; three fourths of them fade away by the seventh week postpartum [4]. This spontaneous regression suggests that they may be permanent structures which are related to the normal vasculature [24]. They rarely disappear completely [39], and they may persist, recur, and enlarge in the same sites during future pregnancies [13,39].

Morphologically and physiologically, the vascular spiders associated with pregnancy are the same as those seen in normal persons and in association with chronic liver disease; however, in chromic liver disease the lesions are usually larger and more abundant [35]. In the absence of hepatic damage, Osler–Weber–Rendu disease is the only significant clinical entity which may be confused [29].

Their presence in pregnancy has always been attributed to high levels of circulating estrogen, and support is given to this by their appearance in women taking oral contraceptives [17, 24]. The liver, which is responsible for the metabolism and excretion of circulation estrogen, is highly burdened in pregnancy, even when not diseased [29]. Indeed, in chronic liver disease, levels of urinary estrogens were found to be increased in a proportion of cases [5]; however, in the case of profuse spider nevi associated with autoimmune hepatitis described by Whiting et al. [36], levels of urinary estrogens were normal [24]. Steroids administered orally led to disappearance of the nevi and improvement in hepatitis [24]. It should be emphasized, however, that no hepatic abnormalities were found in pregnant women with spider angiomata, and they are no more likely to occur in women with toxemia or hypertension [28].

An alternative theory for the formation of spider nevi is the high levels of angiogenesis factors present during pregnancy because of the demands of the vascular placenta. These high levels may incidentally stimulate neovascularization, presenting as vascular spiders, palmar erythema, hemangiomas, and pyogenic granuloma [2, 32, 40].

Treatment should be avoided during pregnancy since, as previously described, many vascular spiders regress postpartum [39]. Nevertheless, not all of them will disappear, and about 10% will persist [10]. On a temporary basis, opaque creams may be used [39]. For insistent patients or persistent lesions, electrodesiccation at low voltage with the use of a fine needle applied to the center of the punctum yields satisfactory cosmetic results [39]. Other treatment modalities include cryosurgery and vascular lasers [28].

5.2
Palmar Erythema

Palmar erythema occurs in 70% of white and 30% of black pregnancies. In the large series by Bean [3] described earlier, he states that 62.5% of whites and 35% of blacks develop palmar erythema when pregnant. Contrary to these high prevalence reports, in a study by Kumari et al. [20], involving 607 pregnant Indian women, no cases of palmar erythema were seen. In addition, in a study by Muzaffar et al. [27] palmar erythema was seen in only 12.1% of cases. This low incidence, like the low incidence of spider nevi, was related to less visibility in darker skin.

The onset of palmar erythema is usually earlier than the onset of vascular spiders, and it typically develops during the first trimester [35, 39]. According to Bean et al. [4], one third of white women developed erythema by the second month of pregnancy. Two forms of palmar erythema were described:

> Bright erythematous areas sharply separated from the bordering normal skin, usually localized to the thenar or hypothenar areas, the palms just proximal to the metacarpophalangeal junction, and the fleshy portion of the tips of the fingers.
> A diffuse mottling of the entire palm with cyanosis and pallor [13, 29, 35, 38, 39]. This form is the more common, and is impossible to differentiate from the palmar erythema seen in hyperthyroidism and hepatic cirrhosis [39].

Palmar erythema fades soon after delivery, usually in 1–2 weeks postpartum [13, 29, 39]. According to Bean et al. [4], 91% had resolution by the seventh week postpartum. For that reason, palmar erythema should not be treated [40]. Though these changes imitate liver disease, it need not be present when they are observed [38]. In addition to liver disease, these clinical findings are similar to palmar erythema found in other conditions such as hyperthyroidism and lupus erythematosus [26].

The fact that both vascular spiders and palmar erythema often occur together in the same patient is significant, and suggests a similar cause. Indeed, it is thought that high levels of circulation estrogenic hormone are also the cause of palmar erythema. Possible contributing factors are the hyperkinetic circulation of the pregnant women, the marked rise in blood volume, and a genetic predisposition [35, 39]. As in spider nevi, there is no association between vascular changes of pregnancy and toxemia or hypertension [3, 4]. Unfortunately, there is no effective treatment [39].

5.3
Hemangiomas

Spontaneous small superficial or subcutaneous cavernous hemangiomas appear at about the third month in less than 5% of pregnancies [13, 39]. They particularly affect the head and neck, but they may also arise on the oral mucosa. [7]. They gradually increase in size until delivery, and then most of them involute completely [13]. The appearance of large hemangiomas with resultant arteriovenous shunting and high-output cardiac failure has been reported [10]. Their cause is unknown [40], and treatment is surgical for persistent lesions [39]. Hemangioendotheliomas and glomangiomas have not unusually developed during pregnancy [39]. Subcutaneous hemangioendotheliomas may occur around the eyes, breasts, or umbilical region and appear as grossly vascular, pigmented, freely movable growths which may have a verrucous appearance and measure up to 6 mm [10]. When they develop, they are often attributed to hormonal influences exerted by the pregnancy [29]. Management is by excision, although, as stated before, the increased vascular state during pregnancy must be taken into consideration [7].

5.4
Cutis Marmorata, Purpura, and Petechia

Cutis marmorata, or "marble skin," of the lower legs, presumably from vasomotor instability secondary to increased estrogen levels, may occur in pregnancy as a transient bluish mottling of the skin on exposure to cold [7, 8, 39]. In a study by Muzaffar et al. [27], cutis marmorata was seen in 0.7% of cases. It usually resolves after delivery [7]. Persistent livedo reticularis postpartum should prompt a search for an underlying cause other than estrogens, such as a collagen vascular disorder, neoplastic disease, or blood dyscrasia [39]. Other manifestations of vascular instability include short episodes of pallor, facial blushing, worsening of preexisting Raynaud's phenomenon, and sensation of heat or cold [19, 26]. Patients also note dermatographism and urticaria, especially during the second half of pregnancy [26].

Purpura and spread petechia are common over the lower extremities, especially during the second half of pregnancy, presumably because of the increased capillary fragility and elevated hydrostatic pressures [7, 26]. The Rumpel–Leede tourniquet testing may be positive in the legs of up to 80% of pregnant women [29]. Usually, both purpura and petechiae spontaneously resolve postpartum [7].

5.5
Edema

Increased capillary permeability, as a result of increased levels of circulating ovarian, placental, and adrenocortical hormones, in addition to sodium and water retention, results in nonpitting edema of the eyelids in about 50% of pregnancies [38, 39]. This edema may also involve the face, hands, ankles, and feet [39]. In a study by Muzaffar et al. [27], 48.5% of patients developed edema. It usually develops during late pregnancy [39]. Edema of the lower extremities not associated with preeclampsia or eclampsia develops in about 70% of pregnancies [39]. This edema is generally apparent in the morning, but improves with activity during the day [39]. Increased hydrostatic pressure in the blood vessels as a result of impairment of blood return because of a gravid uterus is an additional factor causing fluid retention in the lower extremities [16]. Other causes for edema, such as cardiac and renal abnormalities, as well as preeclampsia–eclampsia, need to be excluded [39].

Treatment for the lower extremities includes elevation, sleeping in a Trendelenburg position, and loose clothing [39]. Immersion in water while standing or exercising proved to be of help [25]. Water provides support for the gravid uterus, and it is suggested that the hydrostatic forces may push the extracellular fluid into the venous system, resulting in increased diuresis and subsequent relief of the edema [18]. It was found that water aerobics and static immersion for 30 min led to diuresis of 187 and 180 mL, respectively, which is significantly higher than the diuresis seen after standing on land (65 mL). Standing on land led to a small increase in leg volume compared with water aerobics or static immersion.

The left lateral decubitus position is recommended for reducing impedance in the inferior vena cava, as it was shown that lower-limb perfusion was significantly increased when pregnant women assumed the lateral tilt position [6]. Some investigators advocate well-applied and maintained bandages or stockings [39]. Others have shown no real benefits in the use of elastic supports, and malpositioned or poorly fitting devices can be harmful [14, 15, 34]. According to one study, the optimal pressure for elastic stockings to be used should be 18–8 mmHg, in a graded manner of application [34]. Exercise is another treatment modality which may be of value [39]. A portable external pneumatic intermittent compression device seems to be helpful in reducing peripheral edema and its application for 30 min at 40 Torr to pregnant women, while they were in the left lateral decubitus position, was found to significantly reduce leg volume. This consists of a pump unit connected by flexible tubing with inflatable heavy nylon boots [16]. It should be stressed, however, that all of these measures have been found to be only partially effective [29]. Avoidance of excessive salt intake and, occasionally, treatment with diuretics is recommended [39, 40]. Resolution postpartum almost invariably occurs [39].

5.6 Carpal Tunnel Syndrome

Carpal tunnel syndrome is one of the more common discomforts of pregnancy. The main symptoms include pain, numbness, and swelling of the affected hand, with sparing of the ring finger and little finger [7]. Symptoms are related to compression neuropathy of the median nerve as it passes beneath the flexor retinaculum; characteristically, the attacks are nocturnal [7]. Hormonally mediated retention of salt and water as well as changes in capillary permeability contribute to an increasing soft tissue mass [7]. This condition is difficult to treat during pregnancy but will resolve postpartum [7].

5.7 Varicosities

Varicosities, most frequently involving the saphenous, vulvar, and hemorrhoidal veins, appear in 40% or more of patients (Fig. 5.3) [38, 39]. In a study by Muzaffar et al. [27], varicosities of lower legs were seen in only 2.8% of cases. Raj et al. [31] noted varicose veins in six out of 1,175 women. The low incidence of leg varicosities observed in the study by Muzaffar et al. was attributed to customs and habits of the Lahore women different from those of the Western world. In the Western world, the legs remain in a dependent pose more often than in the Lahore women, who usually work in a sitting position [27].

Hemorrhoidal varicosities may cause pain, discomfort, and bleeding [7, 39]. Varicosities are a well-known result of increased venous pressure in femoral and pelvic vessels caused by the presence of the gravid uterus and increased elastic tissue fragility [38, 39]. The observation that varicosities often appear in the third month of pregnancy (when intrapelvic pressure is not significantly increased) supports the importance of blood vessel

Fig. 5.3 Areas of involvement of varicosities

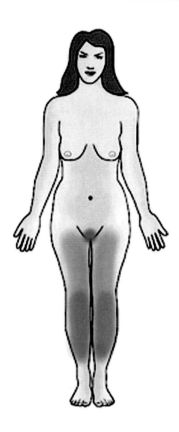

weakness in the formation of dilated veins [39]. In addition, the decreased soft tissue tone in the supporting tissue around the vascular wall also plays a role [29]. A familial tendency to varicose veins and for increased elastic tissue fragility in blood vessels may also be important [39, 40]. Activities that contribute to venous return obstruction, such as prolonged standing and sitting, as well as elastic garters and panty girdles, may be exacerbating factors [39]. Varicosities tend to regress after delivery, but often not completely [39].

In the legs, varicosities may be responsible for pain and, less commonly, thrombosis [29]. Fortunately, thrombosis occurs in less than 10% of pregnant women. This can occur antepartum or postpartum [29], but thromboembolic events are more likely to occur during the first trimester [25]. Levels of circulating coagulation factors such as factors VII, VIII, IX, and X are usually increased [33]. Other severe complications such as thrombophlebitis are quite rare [19]. Hemorrhoids, in contrast to leg varicosities, often produce thrombi during pregnancy [39]. Hemorrhoids can also produce pain and bleeding [29]. Phlegmasia alba dolens, an edematous swelling of the leg following childbirth and due to iliofemoral thrombosis, and phlegmasia cerulean dolens, sudden severe pain, edema, and cyanosis of a limb due to massive venous occlusion, are quite rare [38].

Both vulvar and vaginal varicosities occur and may be symptomatic with pain. Varicosities in the vulva or in the vagina are difficult to treat because it is difficult to provide consistent, firm support to the perineal tissues [29]. Both vaginal and perineal varicosities may also cause difficulties during delivery [29].

The goal of therapy is to collapse the distended superficial veins without impairing the circulation [39]. Measures similar to that for treatment of edema are used to treat leg varicosities: frequent elevation of the legs, sleeping in a Trendelenburg position, lying in a lateral decubitus position, light exercise, avoidance of prolonged sitting and standing, and avoidance of clothing that interferes with venous return should be instituted [14, 29, 39, 40]. Elastic support without restriction for varicose veins in the legs has been advocated [29, 39]. Although these measures are commonly recommended, there are no studies to prove definitively that these measures actually decrease venous hypertension, improve venous return, or decrease the occurrence of varicosities [28]. For persistent leg varicosities, vein stripping, endovascular ablation, endovascular sclerotherapy, or radiofrequency techniques may be beneficial [1]. Supportive panty hose and pressure pads may be used for distended vulvar veins, but their effectiveness is questionable [39]. Hot sitz baths, astringent compresses, laxatives, suppositories, and topical anesthetics are helpful for symptomatic hemorrhoids [39]. Postpartum intervention, such as hemorrhoidectomy, injections of sclerosing agents, and vein strippings, may be indicated for severe and refractory cases [39, 40].

5.8
Pregnancy Gingivitis (Papillomatous Hypertrophy of the Gums, Stomatitis Gravidarum, Hypertrophic Gingivitis of Pregnancy, Marginal Gingivitis)

Between 80 and 100% of pregnant women develop edema and hyperemia of the gums, leading to marginal gingivitis, but with varying degrees of severity [38, 39]. In a study by Kumari et al. [20], gingivitis not attributable to bad oral hygiene was seen in nine out of 607 pregnant women. In a study by Muzaffar et al. [27], 23 out of 140 (16.4%) pregnant women had gingival edema and redness. This discrepancy in prevalence was partially attributed to the rarity of vitamin C deficiency, suggested to be related to gingival changes, in the study population [27].

Pregnancy gingivitis usually appears between the second and fourth months of pregnancy [38]. The clinical picture is identical to that of gingivitis due to other causes [39]. It presents as enlargement and blunting of one or more interdental papillae, generally more marked about the lower front teeth [39]. The gingival margins become glossy, smooth, and swollen, and have a mottled appearance [7, 29, 38, 39]. They appear pink to dark red in color, depending upon the vascularity [38, 39]. They may bleed spontaneously or after minor trauma, and there is associated inflammation, edema, and mild pain [38, 39]. Ulceration is common [39]. Sometimes, generalized gingival hyperplasia may be severe enough to cause chewing, speaking, and breathing problems [12].

Theories for the cause of this condition include local irritative factors, poor oral hygiene (presence of plaque and calculus), and nutritional deficiencies [39]. Indeed, the condition was found to be exacerbated by preexisting peridental diseases [38]. It is suggested that pregnancy does not cause the condition, but altered tissue metabolism in pregnancy accentuates the response to local irritants [12]. Both a deficiency of utilizable estrogen in the gingival tissues and estrogen stimulation have been proposed as causes of the gingivitis [39]. High levels of circulating progesterone are thought to stimulate vascular proliferation at sites of microtrauma [39]. Other causes of gingivitis and gingival enlargement, such as phenytoin and cyclosporine A use as well as myeloproliferative disorders (acute myeloid leukemia), should be excluded [7, 39]. These changes persist throughout pregnancy, increase in severity until the ninth month, and may not regress until 1–2 months after delivery [13, 23]. Epulis nodules may appear on the gums, or preexisting epulis nodules may grow larger [13].

The disease should be managed by appropriate dental hygiene, including plaque and calculus removal, avoidance of trauma, astringents, and use of mouthwashes if inflammation is severe [23, 39]. Therapeutic doses of vitamin C have been advocated [39]. Dental surgery is indicated if chewing causes significant bleeding, or severe ulceration and pain intervenes. Supragingival scaling and subgingival curettage may be helpful [39]. Reassurance constitutes a major part of the treatment, since the majority of lesions regress near term or postpartum, usually in weeks [39].

Paradoxically, despite the apparent inflammation for a prolonged period, pregnancy gingivitis rarely progresses to periodontitis and usually resolves postpartum [25]. With use of cultured human gingival fibroblasts, it was shown that the production of numerous matrix metalloproteinases, responsible for periodontal destruction, was significantly reduced by progesterone [22]. Furthermore, although it is widely believed that pregnancy is harmful to the teeth, studies indicate that the teeth do not soften, and it is mainly the environment of the tooth, namely, the saliva, that is affected [25]. The number of salivary cariogenic microorganisms may increase in pregnancy, at the same time as a decrease in salivary pH and a buffer effect. These changes in salivary composition in late pregnancy and during lactation may in the short term predispose to dental caries and erosion [21].

The nasal mucosa is also often affected, and about 30% of women suffer from nasal symptoms during pregnancy [25]. The hormonal changes occurring during pregnancy favor mucosal edema and relaxation of smooth muscles, thus contributing to nasal congestion [11].

5.9
Granuloma Gravidarum

A lesion similar to a pyogenic granuloma ("pregnancy tumor", pregnancy epulis, pyogenic granuloma of pregnancy or granuloma gravidarum) may develop by proliferation of capillaries within the hypertrophied gum [24, 38]. It has remarkable similarity, both clinically and histologically, to the generic pyogenic granuloma [35, 40]. This lesion usually begins between the second and fifth months of pregnancy in 2–27% of pregnant women, and enlarges continually during the remainder of the gestational period [35, 38, 40]. Raj et al. [31] saw three cases of pyogenic granulomas in their study. It usually occurs in association with extensive gingivitis [38].

Grossly, granuloma gravidarum appears as an oval, friable, smooth, soft or semifirm, pedunculated or sessile, deep-red or purple nodule. It arises from the gingival papilla between adjacent teeth or on the buccal or lingual surface of the marginal gingiva, but it may be attached to the gingiva at any site [29, 35, 38, 40]. It may also be painful, and it bleeds and ulcerates easily when traumatized [29, 35, 38, 40].

Histologically, the lesion consists of granulation tissue which is infiltrated by an inflammatory infiltrate composed of neutrophils, lymphocytes, plasma cells, and histiocytes, covered with stratified squamous epithelium [10, 38].

The cause of the condition is unknown. Theories regarding possible cause relate to hormonal influences on the tissue response to trauma or irritation, such as caries, calculis, and dental crowns [7, 40]. Generally, this tumor is not treated until after delivery because the lesion commonly recedes shortly after parturition, usually several months postpartum, and reassurance of the patient is usually all that is necessary [38, 40].

Maintenance of good oral hygiene may help reduce tumor size [40], and treatment with vitamin C has been advocated [7]. Occasionally a lesion will require excision if size, pain, interference with eating, the patient feels that the cosmetic appearance is too disruptive, or excessive bleeding warrants it [28, 35]. The Nd:YAG laser was used to treat this very vascular lesion, and was preferred over the CO_2 laser because of its superior coagulation characteristics. This technique was suggested to have less risk of bleeding than other surgical techniques [30].

5.10
Unilateral Nevoid Telangiectasia

Unilateral nevoid telangiectasia develops in high estrogen states, such as pregnancy, liver disease related to alcoholism, and end estrogen therapy [1]. Clinically, lesions appear as fine delicate telangiectases mainly located on the upper body in the C3, C4, and trigeminal dermatomes [1]. The distribution may follow Blaschko's lines [1]. Their occurrence during estrogenized states, the dermatoses of distribution, and the presence of anemic halos suggest a relationship with arterial spiders [3, 37]. The telangiectases may clear with decrease in the levels of estrogen [1].

Summary

> Vascular changes are frequent during pregnancy, and occur to a variable extent in all women.

> The main clinical manifestations are spider angiomata and palmar erythema, seen in about 70% of pregnant women. They are thought to be caused by high levels of circulating estrogens and angiogenesis factors. Other contributing factors are the hyperkinetic circulation of the pregnant women, the marked rise in blood volume, and genetic predisposition. They are usually not treated during pregnancy, and resolve postpartum in most cases.

Continued

Summary (continued)

> Varicosities and edema are also very common during pregnancy, and result from increased venous pressure and blood vessel weakening. They are usually managed by conservative therapy such as position changing and exercise. Regression is to be expected after delivery.

> Cutis marmorata may result from vasomotor instability on the legs. Purpura and petechia often occur on the lower extremities as a result of increased hydrostatic pressure and capillary fragility. They usually resolve following delivery.

> The gums may be affected by pregnancy gingivitis, clinically similar to gingivitis due to other causes. Proper dental hygiene is usually all that is needed to treat this condition. Sometimes, granuloma gravidarum, clinically similar to pyogenic granuloma, may develop. This condition also usually resolves after parturition.

References

1. Barankin B, Silver SG, Carruthers A (2002) The skin in pregnancy. J Cutan Med Surg 6:236–240
2. Barnhill RL Wolf JE Jr (1987) Angiogenesis and the skin. J Am Acad Dermatol 16:1226–1242
3. Bean W (1958) Vascular spiders and related lesions of the skin. Thomas, Springfield
4. Bean W, Cogswell R, Dexter M et al (1949) Vascular changes of the skin in pregnancy. Surg Gynecol Obstet 88:739–752
5. Cameron CB (1957) Urinary excretion of oestrone, oestradiol-17beta and oestriol in patients with chronic liver damage. J Endocrinol 15:199–205
6. Downing JW, Bees LT (1976) The influence of lateral tilt on limb blood flow in advanced pregnancy. S Afr Med J 50:728–730
7. Elling SV, Powell FC (1997) Physiological changes in the skin during pregnancy. Clin Dermatol 15:35–43
8. Errickson CV, Matus NR (1994) Skin disorders of pregnancy. Am Fam Physician 49:605–610
9. Esteve E, Saudeau L, Pierre F et al (1994) Physiological cutaneous signs in normal pregnancy: a study of 60 pregnant women. Ann Dermatol Venereol 121:227–231
10. Eudy SF, Baker GF (1990) Dermatopathology for the obstetrician. Clin Obstet Gynecology 33:728–737
11. Gani F, Braida A, Lombardi C et al (2003) Rhinitis in pregnancy. Allerg Immunol (Paris) 35:306–313
12. Gungormus M, Akgul HM, Yilmaz AB et al (2002) Generalized gingival hyperplasia occurring during pregnancy. J Int Med Res 30:353–355
13. Hellreich P (1974) The skin changes of pregnancy. Cutis 13:82–86
14. Husni EA, Ximenes JO, Hamilton FG (1968) Pressure bandaging of the lower extremity. JAMA 206:2715–2718
15. Husni EA, Ximenes JO, Goyette EM (1970) Elastic support of the lower limbs in hospital patients. A critical study. JAMA 214:1456–1462
16. Jacobs MK, McCance KL, Stewart ML (1982) External pneumatic intermittent compression for treatment of dependent pregnancy edema. Nurs Res 31:159–162, 191

17. Jelinek JE (1970) Cutaneous side effects of oral contraceptives. Arch Dermatol 101:181–186
18. Kent T, Gregor J, Deardorff L et al (1999) Edema of pregnancy: a comparison of water aerobics and static immersion. Obstet Gynecol 94:726–729
19. Kroumpouzos G, Cohen LM (2001) Dermatoses of pregnancy. J Am Acad Dermatol 45:1–19; quiz 19–22
20. Kumari R, Jaisankar TJ, Thappa DM (2007) A clinical study of skin changes in pregnancy. Indian J Dermatol Venereol Leprol 73:141
21. Laine MA (2002) Effect of pregnancy on periodontal and dental health. Acta Odontol Scand 60:257–264
22. Lapp CA, Lohse JE, Lewis JB et al (2003) The effects of progesterone on matrix metalloproteinases in cultured human gingival fibroblasts. J Periodontol 74:277–288
23. Martin BJ, Reeb RM (1982) Oral health during pregnancy: a neglected nursing area. MCN Am J Matern Child Nurs 7:391–392
24. McKenzie AW (1971) Skin disorders in pregnancy. Practitioner 206:773–780
25. Muallem MM, Rubeiz NG (2006) Physiological and biological skin changes in pregnancy. Clin Dermatol 24:80–83
26. Murray JC (1990) Pregnancy and the skin. Dermatol Clin 8:327–334
27. Muzaffar F, Hussain I, Haroon TS (1998) Physiologic skin changes during pregnancy: a study of 140 cases. Int J Dermatol 37:429–431
28. Nussbaum R, Benedetto AV (2006) Cosmetic aspects of pregnancy. Clin Dermatol 24:133–141
29. Parmley T, O'Brien TJ (1990) Skin changes during pregnancy. Clin Obstet Gynecol 33:713–717
30. Powell JL, Bailey CL, Coopland AT et al (1994) Nd:YAG laser excision of a giant gingival pyogenic granuloma of pregnancy. Lasers Surg Med 14:178–183
31. Raj S, Khopkar U, Kapasi A et al (1992) Skin in pregnancy. Indian Dermatol Venereol Leprol 58:84–88
32. Rampen FH, Hulsmans RF (1985) Vascular lesions in pregnancy; a hypothesis. J Am Acad Dermatol 12:371–372
33. Richards KA, Stasko T (2002) Dermatologic surgery and the pregnant patient. Dermatol Surg 28:248–256
34. Sigel B, Edelstein AL, Savitch L et al (1975) Type of compression for reducing venous stasis. A study of lower extremities during inactive recumbency. Arch Surg 110:171–175
35. Wade TR, Wade SL, Jones HE (1978) Skin changes and diseases associated with pregnancy. Obstet gynecol 52:233–242
36. Whiting DA, Kallmeyer JC, Simson IW (1970) Widespread arterial spiders in a case of latent hepatitis, with resolution after therapy. Br J Dermatol 82:32–36
37. Wilkin JK, Smith JG Jr, Cullison DA et al (1983) Unilateral dermatomal superficial telangiectasia. Nine new cases and a review of unilateral dermatomal superficial telangiectasia. J Am Acad Dermatol 8:468–477
38. Winton GB, Lewis CW (1982) Dermatoses of pregnancy. J Am Acad Dermatol 6:977–998
39. Wong RC, Ellis CN (1984) Physiologic skin changes in pregnancy. J Am Acad Dermatol 10:929–940
40. Wong RC, Ellis CN (1989) Physiologic skin changes in pregnancy. Semin Dermatol 8:7–11

Physiologic Glandular Changes During Pregnancy

6

Alterations in glandular function during pregnancy are often reported. These alterations include changes in the function of the eccrine glands, apocrine glands, and sebaceous glands.

6.1
Eccrine Glands

Eccrine sweating activity increases progressively near the end of pregnancy [13, 14]. The cause of this change is not certain, but it may be related to increased thyroid activity [13]. During pregnancy, raised thyroid activity and relative iodine deficiency cause the thyroid gland to hypertrophy and to increase its iodine uptake [3]. Others attributed the increased activity to greater weight during pregnancy [14]. In addition, alterations in autonomic nervous system function, producing symptoms and signs of increased vasomotor activity, may result in excess sweating [3, 5]. These physiologic adaptations to pregnancy often result in hyperhidrosis, increased frequency of miliaria, and an increased incidence of dyshidrotic eczema [3]. In a study of 607 pregnant women, however, Kumari et al. [4] reported only 1.65% of pregnant women developing miliaria.

Strangely enough, in the palms, the luteal phase, and to a greater degree pregnancy, is associated with decreased sweating [5]. This has been postulated to be secondary to increased adrenocortical activity, which is responsible for the greater suppression of palmar digital sweating [5].

There is no effective treatment for the increased eccrine sweating [14]. If it is bothersome, a 20% solution of aluminum chloride hexahydrate in ethyl alcohol applied every night for 1 week, and then as necessary, may be effective in many patients [6, 15].

A. Ingber, *Obstetric Dermatology*,
DOI: 10.1007/978-3-540-88399-9, © Springer-Verlag Berlin Heidelberg 2009

6.2
Apocrine Gland

Apocrine gland activity remarkably decreases during pregnancy, temporarily relieving preexisting apocrine gland disorders such as Fox–Fordyce disease and hidradenitis suppurativa [2, 3, 6, 9, 13]. Hidradenitis suppurativa is a chronic relapsing inflammatory skin disease, which characteristically begins after puberty, and is more prevalent in women than in men. This disease affects skin sites with apocrine glands, in particular the axillae and anogenital regions. It is characterized by recurrent abscess formation and draining sinus due to subcutaneous extension with induration, destruction of skin appendages, and ensuing scarring [8]. Fox–Fordyce disease is a chronic disorder of the apocrine glands of the axillae, anogenital, and periareolar regions in women [8]. It should be emphasized, however, that there may be a severe rebound of both diseases postpartum [2, 3, 13]. Hormonal influences probably play a causative role, but there is still debate as to the importance of estrogen, progesterone, and cortisol [2, 14].

6.3
Sebaceous Gland

The effect of pregnancy on sebaceous glands is controversial [9]. Some investigators suggest that sebaceous gland activity generally increases in the second half of pregnancy, with an increased rate of sebum excretion. The peak of symptoms is reached during the third trimester, when complaints of oily skin, especially on the face, are common [3, 14]. Others believe there is no consistent change, with a variable effect on acne [3, 13, 14].

6.3.1
Acne Vulgaris

Most believe that the effect of pregnancy on acne is unpredictable [14]. Acne may develop for the first time during pregnancy, being an early feature of some pregnancies; preexisting acne may be exacerbated; or it may occasionally improve completely [3]. In a study evaluating acne in more than 400 pregnant women, it was found to be improved in 58% of them [10]. After delivery, 75% of women had improvement in acne, 13% had no change, and 12% had worsening of acne [10].

This improvement in acne was associated with therapeutic and beneficial effects of estrogen, which were paralleled by the improvement in acne vulgaris seen with oral contraceptives. Strauss and Pochi [11] reported that ten of 12 female patients who received oral contraceptive pills showed a significant decrease in sebum production. The effect was suggested to be due to the estrogen constituent of the pill. This suppression in sebaceous gland activity was directly correlated with improvement in acne. It was reported that improvement or clearing usually takes about 2 months, but it is not uncommon for a mild flare of acne to be seen in the first month or two of treatment.

In a later study, sebum excretion rates from forehead skin were measured serially during and after pregnancy in ten normal women. In this study, only minor fluctuations occurred during the middle and last trimesters of pregnancy, and there was a pronounced decrease in the postpartum period [1]. Thus, since earlier studies showed that estrogen has an inhibitory effect on the sebaceous glands, it was postulated that during pregnancy either the action of estrogen on the sebaceous glands is blocked or a powerful sebotrophic stimulus is activated [1]. Severe appearance of acne conglobata was reported in a 34-year-old woman 10 days after giving birth. It was suggested, however, that its appearance after delivery might have been coincidental [12].

The unpredictable course of acne during pregnancy was further demonstrated in the study of Muzaffar et al. [7], in which out of the 19 women who had pregnancy-induced changes in acne, 11 (57.9%) noted regression of their disease and eight (42.1%) observed aggravation of the condition.

Acne during pregnancy poses management problems, since a number of systemic anti-acne drugs, ranging from antimicrobials to isotretinoin (13-*cis*-retinoic acid), are contrain-dicated during pregnancy, especially in the first trimester [8].

6.3.2
Breast

Breast changes during pregnancy are numerous, and include enlargement, tenderness, erectile nipples, hyperpigmentation of nipples and areolae, secondary pinkish areolae (arrangement of pale oval areas enclosed in the meshes of a pigmented web), prominence of veins (especially in nulliparous women), striae and Montgomery's tubercles [14]. Mont-gomery's glands or tubercles are hypertrophied sebaceous glands associated with lactiferous ducts on the areolae, and appear in 30–50% of women as multiple small, elevated brown papules during the first trimester, as early as the sixth week of gestation, sufficiently early that they have been considered the first physical sign of pregnancy [3, 6, 9, 14, 15]. In a study of 607 pregnant women, Kumari et al. [4] found that 36.2% had Montgomery's tubercles. They tend to regress postpartum [15].

The causes for all breast changes are likely a combination of increased levels of pituitary, adrenal, placental, and ovarian hormones, with resultant fluid and sodium retention, melanocyte stimulation, and sebaceous gland hyperactivity [14].

Summary

> Alterations in glandular function during pregnancy are common, and include changes in eccrine glands, apocrine glands, and sebaceous glands.
> Eccrine gland activity generally increases during pregnancy, often leading to hyper-hidrosis, miliaria, and dyshidrotic eczema.
> Apocrine gland activity usually decreases during pregnancy, leading to alleviation in Fox–Fordyce disease and hidradenitis suppurativa.
> The effect of pregnancy on sebaceous glands is controversial, and pregnancy has a variable effect on acne.

Continued

6

Summary *Continued*

> Acne may be exacerbated or develop for the first time during pregnancy, or it may occasionally improve completely. Acne during pregnancy poses management problems, since many systemic drugs are contraindicated.
> Sebaceous gland hyperactivity may result in Montgomery's tubercles, hypertrophied sebaceous glands associated with lactiferous ducts on the areolae. They tend to regress postpartum.

References

1. Burton JL, Cunliffe WJ, Millar DG et al (1970) Effect of pregnancy on sebum excretion. Br Med J 2:769–771
2. Cornbleet T (1952) Pregnancy and apocrine gland diseases: hidradenitis, Fox-Fordyce disease. AMA Arch Derm Syphilol 65:12–19
3. Elling SV, Powell FC (1997) Physiological changes in the skin during pregnancy. Clin Dermatol 15:35–43
4. Kumari R, Jaisankar TJ, Thappa DM (2007) A clinical study of skin changes in pregnancy. Indian J Dermatol Venereol Leprol 73:141
5. Mackinnon PC, Mackinnon IL (1955) Palmar sweating in pregnancy. J Obstet Gynaecol Br Emp 62:298–299
6. Martin AG, Leal-Khouri S (1992) Physiologic skin changes associated with pregnancy. Int J Dermatol 31:375–378
7. Muzaffar F, Hussain I, Haroon TS (1998) Physiologic skin changes during pregnancy: a study of 140 cases. Int J Dermatol 37:429–431
8. Oumeish OY, Al-Fouzan AW (2006) Miscellaneous diseases affected by pregnancy. Clin Dermatol 24:113–117
9. Parmley T, O'Brien TJ (1990) Skin changes during pregnancy. Clin Obstet Gynecol 33:713–717
10. Ratzer MA (1964) The influence of marriage, pregnancy and childbirth on acne vulgaris. Br J Dermatol 76:165–168
11. Strauss JS, Pochi PE (1964) Effect of cyclic progestin-estrogen therapy on sebum and acne in women. JAMA 190:815–819
12. van Pelt HP, Juhlin L (1999) Acne conglobata after pregnancy. Acta Derm Venereol 79:169
13. Winton GB, Lewis CW (1982) Dermatoses of pregnancy. J Am Acad Dermatol 6:977–998
14. Wong RC, Ellis CN (1984) Physiologic skin changes in pregnancy. J Am Acad Dermatol 10:929–940
15. Wong RC, Ellis CN (1989) Physiologic skin changes in pregnancy. Semin Dermatol 8:7–11

Inflammatory Skin Conditions During Pregnancy

7.1
Atopic Dermatitis

Atopic dermatitis is an inflammatory itching skin disease, with increasing prevalence worldwide during the last few decades, especially in industrialized countries [43]. One study showed that the cumulative incidence in children born before 1960 was 2–3%, rose to 4–8% during the 1960s, in the 1970s rose to 9–12%, and in the 1980s rose to 15–20% [57] Atopic dermatitis has a variable course with regard to age, morphology, and distribution [42], and it is more frequently reported by women than by men, with the highest rate (25.3%) seen in the age range of 20–29 years [43].

Atopic dermatitis is considered to be a multifactorial disease influenced by genetic predisposition and environmental factors. The process of this inflammatory condition was suggested to be dependent on the production of cytokines by allergen-specific Th2 cells [35]. This theory was recently further strengthened by showing that transgenic mice expressing high levels of Th2 cytokines developed diffuse spontaneous atopic dermatitis and expressed high levels of serum IgE [35]. Pregnancy, as described earlier, is also suggested to be a Th2 condition [70]. Thus, it would be expected that atopic dermatitis would flare during pregnancy [62].

Atopic dermatitis is considered to be quite common during pregnancy, affecting 72 out of 200 pregnant women presenting to a specialty clinic for pregnancy dermatoses in one prospective study [64]. However, it should be taken into account that atopic dermatitis is highly prevalent in the general population and the bias of a referral center [62]. In addition, atopic dermatitis was traditionally considered to worsen in most pregnant women and improve in only a few patients [47]. However, when patients with atopic dermatitis were asked to assess the course of their disease during pregnancy in a retrospective study of 50 women, with a total of 88 full-term pregnancies, variability was typical. Twenty-six women (52%) reported a deterioration in their skin during pregnancy, whereas improvement was noted by 12 women (24%). No change was noted in 12 women (24%) [29]. It should be noted that the exacerbation may be partially attributed to the pruritus of pregnancy [47].

A. Ingber, *Obstetric Dermatology*,
DOI: 10.1007/978-3-540-88399-9, © Springer-Verlag Berlin Heidelberg 2009

7

The variable influence of pregnancy on atopic dermatitis is a key example for the intricacy of the pregnancy–disease interaction, and lends further support for the hypothesis that the Th2 paradigm of pregnancy is out of date and an oversimplification [14, 62].

The gestation stage at which deterioration occurs is also debatable. One study found that the incidence decreases with the advancement of pregnancy – out of 29 pregnancies, there was worsening of atopic dermatitis in the first 10 weeks in nine pregnancies, between 10 and 20 weeks in a further 12 pregnancies, between 20 and 30 weeks in four pregnancies, and only in one pregnancy between 30 weeks and term. In three others a fare-up of the skin occurred in the puerperium [29]. However, a study by Vaughan et al. [64] found that the gestation at presentation varied throughout all three trimesters, when out of 72 pregnant women 17 women presented in the first, 32 in the second, and 23 in the third trimester. Surprisingly, though the pregnant patients in this study had typical eczematous clinical features, serum IgE levels were elevated in only 13 women.

Exacerbation of dermatitis was also seen in 33% of female patients suffering from atopic dermatitis in the premenstrual period. Thus, the phenomenon of flaring of atopic dermatitis during the premenstrual period and during pregnancy strongly suggests an influence of the increased serum progesterone levels and other female sex hormones on skin sensitivity [29, 64].

Recently, it was suggested that changes in filaggrin, a key protein that facilitates terminal differentiation of the epidermis and formation of the skin barrier, are very strong predisposing factors for atopic dermatitis [48]. It was shown that the null variant of filaggrin is associated with a 7.7 odds ratio to develop atopic dermatitis [3]. It is still unknown, however, whether such changes occur during pregnancy [69].

Breast-feeding is often a problem for women with atopic dermatitis due to nipple eczematization. There is also a problem postpartum with irritant hand dermatitis, owing to increased exposure to such common irritants as food or detergents [47].

Flares of atopic dermatitis during pregnancy are not known to cause adverse fetal outcome [62]. In addition, with the exception of infected dermatitis, the condition should not affect a woman's birth plan or her obstetric outcome after delivery [69]. However, atopic dermatitis in the mother is a known risk factor for atopy in a child. It was found that the odds ratio for atopic dermatitis between mothers and siblings is 2.66 relative to that of a control [16].

Recommendations for treatment of atopic dermatitis during pregnancy should emphasize the role of emollients as an integral part of the treatment, since they can be used safely during pregnancy. Topical steroids can be used during pregnancy relatively safely, except for very potent ones [69]. When dermatitis remains despite optimization of topical steroids, narrowband UVB has been suggested to be the safest second-line treatment in pregnancy [69].

7.2
Psoriasis

Psoriasis is a common papulosquamous disease affecting 1–3% of the population, and accounts for nearly 5% of all skin diseases [36, 41, 60]. It may cause considerable morbidity and occupational disability. There seems to be a gender difference, although women generally develop the disease earlier than men [60, 69]. Psoriasis has a genetic component; however, the mode of inheritance is not well understood. There is a bimodal age distribution, with peaks in the third and fifth decades. Known precipitating factors include stress, infection, trauma, and drug therapy.

The course of psoriasis during pregnancy is unpredictable and only a few controlled studies have examined this relationship [9]. However, from review of the available studies, it seems that during pregnancy, if psoriasis alters, it is more likely to improve than worsen, and the number of patients whose psoriasis improves during pregnancy is approximately double the number of patients whose psoriasis worsens during pregnancy [17, 45]. Major studies that checked the changes in psoriasis during pregnancy are summarized in Tables 7.1 and 7.2.

Most women report gradual improvement, but the improvement may also be abrupt [9]. If improvement occurs, it is more likely to occur during the first trimester [9, 44]. If exacerbation occurs, it is also more likely to be progressive over the course of pregnancy, but some report sudden worsening [9]. Onset of exacerbation is more common during the first trimester than during the third one [44].

If psoriasis changes in the postpartum period, it is much more likely to deteriorate than improve [17]. Table 7.3 summarizes the major studies examining this aspect. Of those patients whose psoriasis worsened postpartum, the majority noticed improvement during pregnancy [44].

Table 7.1 Effect of pregnancy on psoriasis. Distributed by number of patients

No. of women	Improved	Unchanged	Deteriorated	Reference
60	25	27	8	[17]
300	150	69	81	[22]
1,018	326	509	183	[21]
82	34	34	14	[10]
85	36	33	16	[49]
63	15	41	7	[33]
70	27	40	3	[36]
90	57	21	12	[9]
46	17	21	8	[44]
47	26	10	11	[45]
1,861	713	805	343	

Table 7.2 Effect of pregnancy on psoriasis. Distributed by number of pregnancies

No. of women	Improved	Unchanged	Deteriorated	Reference
110	46	48	16	[17]
204	33	147	24	[33]
91	51	16	24	[53]
405	130	211	64	

Table 7.3 Changes in psoriasis status after pregnancy

No. of women	Improved	Unchanged	Deteriorated	Reference
60	7	18	35	[17]
90	0	11	79	[9]
46	2	25	19	[44]
47	4	12	31	[45]
243	13	66	164	

The age of the patient and the type or severity of the disease is not associated with improvement or deterioration of psoriasis [44]. The gender of the fetus also does not have a demonstrable effect on the type of change seen during pregnancy [44].

The effects of pregnancy on psoriasis are often consistent in the same woman [44, 47, 53]; however, improvement in one gestation is not an indication that successive gestations will achieve the same results [33, 36]. In addition, few patients may note both an improvement and a worsening during the same pregnancy [9]. No relationship was observed between the severity of the psoriasis and the incidence of remission as an outcome of pregnancy [53].

Major hormonal changes appear to have some effect on psoriasis, and women frequently report that menopause is associated with exacerbation of psoriasis. This is in agreement with the bimodal age of onset of the disease (around the age of 55). However, no effect on psoriasis was seen with the menstrual cycle, fertility drugs, and oral contraceptive pills [44].

As noted earlier, pregnancy is a condition in which the immunologic activity is suppressed, in order to accept the fetus as a foreign antigen. This activity is increased in the postpartum period [28]. These immunologic changes are probably modulated by hormonal changes [9]. Estrogens have been shown to encourage B-cell immunity but to suppress T-cell-mediated immunity [45]. Progesterone was suggested to have an even more profound effect, and to be mainly immunosuppressive [44, 45]. Progesterone exerts its effect by downregulating T-cell proliferative response, and it has been shown by animal studies to be the key factor in uterine immunosuppression, by causing a delay of rejection of allografts placed in the uterus [44, 45]. Recently, however, it was shown that progesterone levels alone did not correlate with changes in psoriasis, but rather increased estrogen levels, and especially increased levels of estrogen relative to those of progesterone [45]. Other hormones suggested to play a role are human placental lactogen and human chorionic gonadotropin; however, their role is not well defined [44].

It was suggested that the high levels of IL-10 in pregnancy, probably the result of the maternal decidual cells production [63], may also add to the favorable effect of pregnancy on the course of the disease [32].

The hormonal changes, in addition to the immunologic changes, may also directly affect keratinocytes. Studies have shown that skin cells metabolize steroid hormones, specifically estrogen and progesterone [40, 71]. There is still no evidence, however, that they might slow keratinocyte growth other than indirectly through an immune-mediated event [9].

It is well known that stress may lead to exacerbation of psoriasis, and such emotional changes may thus affect the course of this disease. One study indeed elicited comments from several patients substantiating this point; however, these variables are extremely difficult to qualify [9].

It is advised to induce a period of remission or to optimize control of psoriasis before conception to help minimize exacerbations during pregnancy [68]. This may require revision of the therapeutic approach, particularly in cases of severe disease [60]. It is recommended to avoid all medication during pregnancy, and rely on conservative treatment [60].

Topical treatments are first-line treatments in psoriasis, and emollients, topical corticosteroids, and topically applied calcipotriene, anthralin, and tacrolimus appear to be safe choices for control of localized psoriasis in pregnancy [60, 68]. The safety of using coal tar products during pregnancy is unclear, although such products are probably safe during the second and third trimesters [68]. For widespread psoriasis during pregnancy, UVB treatment seems to be the safest option, especially when topical application of other agents is not practical [60]. In cases of severe psoriasis that is recalcitrant to topical or UVB treatment, short-term use of cyclosporine during pregnancy is probably the safest option [60].

Pregnancy was suggested to be a risk factor for developing psoriatic arthritis, and 30% of women with psoriatic arthritis associate the onset of their disease with the postpartum period [37]. In that study, there was no evidence that pregnancy influenced the onset of the rash; therefore, in some women pregnancy is a trigger for onset of arthritis but not for skin psoriasis [37]. In the same study, there was a temporal relationship between the onset of arthritis and the menopause, another time at which there are major hormonal changes. Thus, it was suggested that hormonal changes may be a factor in determining the onset of psoriatic arthritis [37]. However, it was also reported that established psoriatic arthritis may improve during pregnancy [38, 60].

Psoriasis does not affect fertility or rates of miscarriages, birth defects, or premature birth, and having psoriasis should not affect the timing or mode of delivery [58]. However, it should be again stressed that many treatments for psoriasis are associated with potential problems during pregnancy [68]. Psoriasis can localize into scars (Koebner's phenomenon), but this phenomenon has not been reported in perineal scars, although theoretically it can occur at any site of epidermal injury [68]. The risk of infection and delayed healing of cesarean section wounds is theoretically higher, but no studies have examined this risk [54].

7.3
Urticaria

Urticaria consists of circumscribed, raised, pruritic, and erythematous lesions caused by edema involving the superficial dermis. Symptoms persisting for less than 6 weeks are termed "acute," and those persisting longer are considered chronic [56]. Angioedema refers to deeper areas of the dermis, subcutaneous tissue, or submucosa [56].

Urticaria or angioedema may occur during pregnancy from any of the causes, agents, and medications noted in the nonpregnant state or may be restricted to pregnancy, redeveloping in subsequent pregnancies [56].

Chronic pregnancy-associated urticaria or angioedema syndrome was reported in three out of 554 consecutive patients with urticaria [13]. The cause of this syndrome is uncertain, but some observations suggest possible allergic sensitization to endogenous hormones, particularly progesterone [56]. This assumption is supported by the findings of Farah and Shbaklu [20], who reported two patients with urticaria occurring at the mid- and premenstrual part of the cycle. The lesions were exacerbated with progesterone injection, there were positive skin reactions to progesterone, passive transfer of serum into normal subjects with prepared sites tested to progesterone elicited wheals, and immunofluorescence of antibodies reactive to the luteinizing cells of the corpus luteum was demonstrated. This is a case of autoimmune progesterone dermatitis, which can, among others, be characterized by urticarial lesions. In addition, endogenous progesterone has been implicated as a cause of recurrent anaphylaxis [39].

7.4
Hereditary Angioedema

Hereditary angioneuritic edema (HAE) is an infrequent autosomal dominant disorder caused by a deficiency or malfunction of C1-esterase inhibitor, which, when normally present, functions to inhibit the first component of the complement cascade. Clinical symptoms and signs of HAE include recurrent 1–4-day attacks of nonpruritic and nonurticarial angioedema of the extremities, abdomen, face, and, potentially most seriously, larynx. It is assumed that the lack of normal C1-esterase inhibitor function to modulate an activated complement cascade leads to increased function of kinin-like fragments and other pharmacologically active mediators. Episodes generally are sporadic but often are triggered by trauma, stress, infections, and extreme temperature fluctuations [56].

In a series of 73 affected persons, Frank et al. [24] reported that five out of 12 women had an increase in attacks during their menstrual periods; however, only one of four who were menopausal reported any improvement in the disease. The association between disease activity and menstruation was also found by other investigators [6]. The effect of pregnancy as reported by Frank et al. [24] was remarkably better. Among ten women with a total of 25 pregnancies, none had an attack of angioedema at delivery despite the trauma to the birth canal. In 23 of 25 pregnancies, the women had noticeably fewer or no attacks in the last two trimesters. Interestingly, two young women reported greater frequency and severity of attacks while using oral contraceptives of the combined estrogen–progesterone type.

Although pregnancy generally appears to produce a remarkable calming effect on HAE, there are reports of exacerbations during pregnancy. One woman experienced worsening of HAE during three pregnancies [67]. In addition, postpartum exacerbations have been reported [67]. One maternal death after delivery occurred from localized perineal swelling with secondary irreversible shock [51]. The relationship between progesterone levels and HAE attacks was proved by the study of Visy et al. [65], who showed that the attack rate was 5 times higher in women with high progesterone levels than in women with normal or low serum concentrations. The difference was even higher when only subcutaneous attacks were considered. According to their data, a high variability was noted in the incidence of attacks during pregnancy – out of 25 pregnant patients, pregnancy was associated with a higher incidence of attacks in 36%; edema formation was less common in 56%, and 8% experienced no change in the frequency of symptoms.

Recently, a unique estrogen-dependent variant of inherited angioedema with normal C1-esterase inhibitor level and function was described. The clinical manifestations are identical to the classic forms of HAE, except that the symptoms are dependent on relatively high estrogen levels, whether endogenous (pregnancy) or exogenous (oral contraceptives, hormone replacement therapy, or both) in origin [5].

Ideally, all prophylactic drugs should be stopped during pregnancy, and, if possible, before conception. If prophylaxis is required, tranexamic acid at standard doses should be used [23]. Severe attacks during pregnancy should be treated with concentrate as in the nonpregnant patient. Replacement with C1-esterase inhibitor concentrate is the most effective treatment of HAE and can be used at any period of pregnancy. In high-risk patients, it can be given in regular intervals throughout the pregnancy [12, 27].

Vaginal delivery does not require special measures; there may be local swelling of the vulva and infusion sites but this will usually resolve without involvement. If an operative delivery is required, regional analgesia should be used [23].

Involvement of the bowel wall typically causes severe abdominal colic, vomiting, and guarding without fever, leukocytosis, elevated sedimentation rate, or rigidity [56]: therefore, abdominal pain must be carefully evaluated since hasty surgical intervention will possibly trigger a systemic attack [18]. A thorough history and complete physical examination are necessary to differentiate surgical or obstetric causes of severe abdominal pain in these patients [18].

7.5
Erythema Nodosum

Erythema nodosum (EN) is a well-known self-limited condition, characterized by the occurrence of tender, nonsuppurative, slightly raised, red, inflammatory nodules, mostly localized on the extensor sides of the lower part of the legs and forearms [19, 34, 55]. Lesions are sometimes associated with fever, swelling of the legs, and arthralgia [55]. There is a predominance of the female sex in the reproductive age [34]. EN is probably a hypersensitivity reaction, mediated by immune mechanisms, characterized by inflammatory nodules in the dermis and subcutaneous tissue [7, 15]. It is regarded as secondary to a variety of underlying disorders, especially bacterial (streptococcal, mycobacterial: tuberculosis and leprosy, yersinia), fungal and viral infections, internal disease (sarcoidosis, ulcerative colitis, Behçet's syndrome, lupus erythematosus, etc.), and drug reactions (sulfonamides, oral contraceptives), but many occur cases in pregnancy without an underlying cause being found [15, 34].

The prevalence was given as 2.4 per 10,000 population per year [34]. Its incidence varies in different countries; the condition constitutes less than 0.5% of cases seen in private or clinical practice [34].

EN is characterized histopathologically by a septal panniculitis in which the fibrous septa of subcutaneous fat become inflamed. Lipocytes ordinarily are spared, but adjacent fat necrosis has been noted [11].

The time of appearance of EN during pregnancy is usually during the first trimester, but it may occur also near the end of pregnancy (Table 7.4).

Table 7.4 Time of appearance of erythema nodosum during pregnancy

No. of women	I	II	III	Reference
1	–	1	–	[46]
19	17	2	–	[26]
1	–	–	1	[15]
1	1	–	–	[72]
1	1	–	–	[7]
4	1	3	–	[34]
2	1	1	–	[25]
4	3	–	1	[55]
8	5	3	–	[52]
3	2	–	1	[61]
3	3	–	–	[59]
47	34	10	3	

The influence of female sex hormones on EN has been known for a very long time [26]. The observation that pregnancy may form an etiologic basis for the occurrence of EN may be strengthened by the fact that EN can be provoked by contraceptive agents [34]. However, estrogens or progesterones alone were unable to cause EN, but only the combination of estrogens and progesterones was causative [34]. It is believed that oral contraceptives and pregnancy do not cause EN but that they produce a hormonal environment that is more suitable for those factors or agents that cause the disorder [4]. It may be that a specific relative level of the two hormones may be required. This may explain why EN during pregnancy is almost always encountered in the first half of gestation; this may be the only time during pregnancy when the necessary hormonal environment is present [4].

Stein et al. [59] reported three women with EN appearing in the first trimester. In all cases, the father of the fetus differed from the father of the fetus in previous pregnancies. This suggests that paternal antigens may be important in the pathogenesis of EN occurring in pregnant women. Expression of paternal antigens in fetal tissue may trigger the immune response of EN in a woman immunologically primed by pregnancy.

The condition is a self-limited condition, requiring at most such symptomatic treatment as bed rest and pain-relieving medication [34]. No adverse effect on maternal or fetal systems should be anticipated [34].

7.6
Contact Dermatitis

Allergic contact dermatitis is a classic type 1 cytokine-dominated immune reaction [2]; thus, in pregnancy, this Th1-mediated condition is expected to be ameliorated. In addition, the high levels of IL-10 observed during pregnancy are also expected to improve this condition, and it has already been shown that the administration of IL-10 blocks the effector phase in allergic contact hypersensitivity reactions [30, 31].

Nevertheless, clinical data on the influence of the menstrual cycle or pregnancy on cutaneous reactivity continues to be confusing, inconclusive, and hypothetical [50]. One study evaluating 505 pregnant patients seen in two dermatology hospitals found that contact dermatitis was a relatively common condition, with 11 patients (2%) reporting contact dermatitis [1]. Changes, if they occur at all, would appear to be premenstrual or in the third trimester of pregnancy [50]. The hormonal effects on contact dermatitis were evaluated in several studies, and it was found that during the follicular phase of the cycle there seems to be an inhibition of the eliciting phase of allergic contact dermatitis; this was suggested to be due to estradiol-induced inhibition of delayed hypersensitivity type reactions [8].

Our experience shows that many women have exacerbation of symptoms or experience the first appearance of this condition after delivery. Postpartum, the immunologic milieu is biased toward Th1, a tendency that may explain the exacerbation of contact dermatitis, being a Th1-mediated condition.

It is usually not advised to perform patch testing in pregnant women. Although the small amounts of allergens are not expected to affect the fetus, in the case of an unwanted event during pregnancy or delivery this test could be blamed by the mother or her surrounding environment [66].

Summary

> *Atopic dermatitis*, although traditionally considered to worsen during pregnancy, is probably variably affected. Nipple eczematization and irritant hand dermatitis are common postpartum. Although flares of atopic dermatitis during pregnancy are not known to cause adverse fetal outcome, atopic dermatitis in the mother is a known risk factor for atopy in a child. First-line treatment is topical corticosteroids and emollients, followed by UVB treatment.

> *Psoriasis* is probably more likely to improve than worsen during pregnancy, but postpartum it usually worsens. It is advised to optimize control of psoriasis before conception. Topical treatments are first-line therapy during pregnancy, followed by UVB treatment for generalized disease.

> *Urticaria* may occur during pregnancy from the usual causes, but also without any trigger.

> *Hereditary angioneuritic edema* is usually remarkably better during pregnancy, but variability is common. Vaginal delivery does not usually require special measures.

> *Erythema nodosum* may appear during pregnancy, usually during the first trimester, probably as a result of specific relative levels of estrogen and progesterone. Since the condition is self-limited, no treatment is usually required.

> *Contact dermatitis* appears to be exacerbated during the premenstrual period or in the third trimester of pregnancy. It is usually not advised to perform patch testing in pregnant women.

7

References

1. Ambros-Rudolph CM, Mullegger RR, Vaughan-Jones SA et al (2006) The specific dermatoses of pregnancy revisited and reclassified: results of a retrospective two-center study on 505 pregnant patients. J Am Acad Dermatol 54:395–404
2. Asadullah K, Sabat R, Wiese A et al (1999) Interleukin-10 in cutaneous disorders: implications for its pathophysiological importance and therapeutic use. Arch Dermatol Res 291:628–636
3. Barker JN, Palmer CN, Zhao Y et al (2007) Null mutations in the filaggrin gene (FLG) determine major susceptibility to early-onset atopic dermatitis that persists into adulthood. J Invest Dermatol 127:564–567
4. Bartelsmeyer JA, Petrie RH (1990) Erythema nodosum, estrogens, and pregnancy. Clin Obstet Gynecol 33:777–781
5. Binkley KE, Davis A 3rd (2000) Clinical, biochemical, and genetic characterization of a novel estrogen-dependent inherited form of angioedema. J Allergy Clin Immunol 106:546–550
6. Blohme G, Ysander L, Korsan-Bengtsen K et al (1972) Hereditary angioneurotic oedema in three families. Symptomatic heterogeneity, complement analysis and therapeutic trials. Acta Med Scand 191:209–219
7. Bombardieri S, Munno OD, Di Punzio C et al (1977) Erythema nodosum associated with pregnancy and oral contraceptives. Br Med J 1:1509–1510
8. Bonamonte D, Foti C, Antelmi AR et al (2005) Nickel contact allergy and menstrual cycle. Contact Dermatitis 52:309–313
9. Boyd AS, Morris LF, Phillips CM et al (1996) Psoriasis and pregnancy: hormone and immune system interaction. Int J Dermatol 35:169–172
10. Braun-Falco O, Burg G, Farber EM (1972) Psoriasis. A questionnaire study of 536 patients. Munch Med Wochenschr 114:1105–1110
11. Brodell RT, Mehrabi D (2000) Underlying causes of erythema nodosum. Lesions may provide clue to systemic disease. Postgrad Med 108:147–149
12. Caliskaner Z, Ozturk S, Gulec M et al (2007) A successful pregnancy and uncomplicated labor with C1INH concentrate prophylaxis in a patient with hereditary angioedema. Allergol Immunopathol (Madr) 35:117–119
13. Champion RH, Roberts SO, Carpenter RG et al (1969) Urticaria and angio-oedema. A review of 554 patients. Br J Dermatol 81:588–597
14. Chaouat G, Ledee-Bataille N, Dubanchet S et al (2004) TH1/TH2 paradigm in pregnancy: paradigm lost? Cytokines in pregnancy/early abortion: reexamining the TH1/TH2 paradigm. Int Arch Allergy Immunol 134:93–119
15. Daw E (1971) Recurrent erythema nodosum of pregnancy. Br Med J 2:44
16. Diepgen TL, Blettner M (1996) Analysis of familial aggregation of atopic eczema and other atopic diseases by odds ratio regression models. J Invest Dermatol 106:977–981
17. Dunna SF, Finlay AY (1989) Psoriasis: improvement during and worsening after pregnancy. Br J Dermatol 120:584
18. Duvvur S, Khan F, Powell K (2007) Hereditary angioedema and pregnancy. J Matern Fetal Neonatal Med 20:563–565
19. Eudy SF, Baker GF (1990) Dermatopathology for the obstetrician. Clin Obstet Gynecol 33:728–737
20. Farah FS, Shbaklu Z (1971) Autoimmune progesterone urticaria. J Allergy Clin Immunol 48:257–261
21. Farber EM, Nall ML (1974) The natural history of psoriasis in 5,600 patients. Dermatologica 148:1–18

22. Farber EM, Bright RD, Nall ML (1968) Psoriasis. A questionnaire survey of 2,144 patients. Arch Dermatol 98:248–259
23. Fay A, Abinun M (2002) Current management of hereditary angio-oedema (C'1 esterase inhibitor deficiency). J Clin Pathol 55:266–270
24. Frank MM, Gelfand JA, Atkinson JP (1976) Hereditary angioedema: the clinical syndrome and its management. Ann Intern Med 84:580–593
25. Gordon H (1961) Erythema nodosum. A review of one hundred and fifteen cases. Br J Dermatol 73:393–409
26. Hannuksela M, Ahvonen P (1969) Erythema nodosum due to Yersinia enterocolitica. Scand J Infect Dis 1:17–19
27. Hermans C (2007) Successful management with C1-inhibitor concentrate of hereditary angioedema attacks during two successive pregnancies: a case report. Arch Gynecol Obstet 276:271–276
28. Iwatani Y, Amino N, Tachi J et al (1988) Changes of lymphocyte subsets in normal pregnant and postpartum women: postpartum increase in NK/K (Leu 7) cells. Am J Reprod Immunol Microbiol 18:52–55
29. Kemmett D, Tidman MJ (1991) The influence of the menstrual cycle and pregnancy on atopic dermatitis. Br J Dermatol 125:59–61
30. Kondo S, McKenzie RC, Sauder DN (1994) Interleukin-10 inhibits the elicitation phase of allergic contact hypersensitivity. J Invest Dermatol 103:811–814
31. Kotenko SV, Krause CD, Izotova LS et al (1997) Identification and functional characterization of a second chain of the interleukin-10 receptor complex. EMBO J 16:5894–5903
32. Kroumpouzos G, Cohen LM (2001) Dermatoses of pregnancy. J Am Acad Dermatol 45:1–19; quiz 19–22
33. Lane C, Crawford G (1937) Psoriasis: a statistical study of 231 cases. Arch Dermatol Chic 35:1051–1061
34. Langer R, Bukovsky I, Lipshitz I et al (1979) Erythema nodosum associated with pregnancy. Case reports. Eur J Obstet Gynecol Reprod Biol 9:399–401
35. Lee GR, Flavell RA (2004) Transgenic mice which overproduce Th2 cytokines develop spontaneous atopic dermatitis and asthma. Int Immunol 16:1155–1160
36. Lomholt G (1963) Psoriasis: prevalence, spontaneous course, and genetics: a census study on the prevalence of skin diseases on the Faroe Islands. Gad, Copenhagen
37. McHugh NJ, Laurent MR (1989) The effect of pregnancy on the onset of psoriatic arthritis. Br J Rheumatol 28:50–52
38. McNeill ME (1988) Multiple pregnancy-induced remissions of psoriatic arthritis: case report. Am J Obstet Gynecol 159:896–897
39. Meggs WJ, Pescovitz OH, Metcalfe D et al (1984) Progesterone sensitivity as a cause of recurrent anaphylaxis. N Engl J Med 311:1236–1238
40. Milewich L, Shaw CB, Sontheimer RD (1988) Steroid metabolism by epidermal keratinocytes. Ann N Y Acad Sci 548:66–89
41. Mitchel J (1967) Proportionate distribution of skin diseases in a dermatological practice: enumeration by standard nomenclature of 12,578 cases from clinic and private practice. Can Med Assoc J 97:1346
42. Mohrenschlager M, Darsow U, Schnopp C et al (2006) Atopic eczema: what's new? J Eur Acad Dermatol Venereol 20:503–511, 513; quiz 512
43. Montnemery P, Nihlen U, Goran Lofdahl C et al (2003) Prevalence of self-reported eczema in relation to living environment, socio-economic status and respiratory symptoms assessed in a questionnaire study. BMC Dermatol 3:4
44. Mowad CM, Margolis DJ, Halpern AC et al. (1998) Hormonal influences on women with psoriasis. Cutis 61:257–260

45. Murase JE, Chan KK, Garite TJ et al (2005) Hormonal effect on psoriasis in pregnancy and post partum. Arch Dermatol 141:601–606
46. Nilehn B, Sjostrom B, Damgaard K et al (1968) Yersinia enterocolitica in patients with symptoms of infectious disease. Acta Pathol Microbiol Scand 74:101–113
47. Oumeish OY, Al-Fouzan AW (2006) Miscellaneous diseases affected by pregnancy. Clin Dermatol 24:113–117
48. Palmer CN, Irvine AD, Terron-Kwiatkowski A et al (2006) Common loss-of-function variants of the epidermal barrier protein filaggrin are a major predisposing factor for atopic dermatitis. Nat Genet 38:441–446
49. Park BS, Youn JI (1998) Factors influencing psoriasis: an analysis based upon the extent of involvement and clinical type. J Dermatol 25:97–102
50. Patil S, Maibach HI (1994) Effect of age and sex on the elicitation of irritant contact dermatitis. Contact Dermatitis 30:257–264
51. Postnikoff IM, Pritzker KP (1979) Hereditary angioneurotic edema: an unusual case of maternal mortality. J Forensic Sci 24:473–478
52. Psychos DN, Voulgari PV, Skopouli FN et al (2000) Erythema nodosum: the underlying conditions. Clin Rheumatol 19:212–216
53. Raychaudhuri SP, Navare T, Gross J et al (2003) Clinical course of psoriasis during pregnancy. Int J Dermatol 42:518–520
54. Saini R, Shupack JL (2003) Psoriasis: to cut or not to cut, what say you? Dermatol Surg 29:735–740
55. Salvatore MA, Lynch PJ (1980) Erythema nodosum, estrogens, and pregnancy. Arch Dermatol 116:557–558
56. Schatz M, Zeiger RS (1997) Asthma and allergy in pregnancy. Clin Perinatol 24:407–432
57. Schultz Larsen F, Diepgen T, Svensson A (1996) The occurrence of atopic dermatitis in north Europe: an international questionnaire study. J Am Acad Dermatol 34:760–764
58. Seeger JD, Lanza LL, West WA et al (2007) Pregnancy and pregnancy outcome among women with inflammatory skin diseases. Dermatology 214:32–39
59. Stein DH, Lee RV, Paul JJ et al (1988) Erythema nodosum. J Allergy Clin Immunol 81:761
60. Tauscher AE, Fleischer AB Jr, Phelps KC et al (2002) Psoriasis and pregnancy. J Cutan Med Surg 6:561–570
61. Tay YK (2000) Erythema nodosum in Singapore. Clin Exp Dermatol 25:377–380
62. Torgerson RR, Marnach ML, Bruce AJ et al (2006) Oral and vulvar changes in pregnancy. Clin Dermatol 24:122–132
63. Trautman MS, Collmer D, Edwin SS et al (1997) Expression of interleukin-10 in human gestational tissues. J Soc Gynecol Invest 4:247–253
64. Vaughan Jones SA, Hern S, Nelson-Piercy C et al (1999) A prospective study of 200 women with dermatoses of pregnancy correlating clinical findings with hormonal and immunopathological profiles. Br J Dermatol 141:71–81
65. Visy B, Fust G, Varga L et al (2004) Sex hormones in hereditary angioneurotic oedema. Clin Endocrinol (Oxf) 60:508–515
66. Wahlberg J, Lindberg M (2006) Patch testing. Springer, Berlin
67. Warin RP, Cunliffe WJ, Greaves MW et al (1986) Recurrent angioedema: familial and oestrogen-induced. Br J Dermatol 115:731–734
68. Weatherhead S, Robson SC, Reynolds NJ (2007) Management of psoriasis in pregnancy. BMJ 334:1218–1220
69. Weatherhead S, Robson SC, Reynolds NJ (2007) Eczema in pregnancy. BMJ 335:152–154

70. Wegmann TG, Lin H, Guilbert L et al (1993) Bidirectional cytokine interactions in the maternal-fetal relationship: is successful pregnancy a TH2 phenomenon? Immunol Today 14:353–356
71. Weinstein GD, Frost P, Hsia SL (1968) In vitro interconversion of estrone and 17-beta-estradiol in human skin and vaginal mucosa. J Invest Dermatol 51:4–10
72. Wetherill JH (1971) Recurrent erythema nodosum of pregnancy. Br Med J 3:535

8.1
Systemic Lupus Erythematosus

Systemic lupus erythematosus (SLE) is a relatively common disease, with an incidence of approximately one per 1,000 women [41]. The mean onset of disease is about 30 years of age [15]; therefore, it is not surprising that SLE and pregnancy may occur coincidentally together, and indeed lupus is seen in approximately one of every 1,660 pregnancies [45].

There is an abundance of material published on SLE in pregnancy; however, despite this vast amount of literature, there is no agreement regarding the effects of pregnancy on SLE clinical manifestations, or whether there are adverse effects of SLE on fetal or maternal outcome [15].

Fertility is generally considered not to be affected by SLE. It might be present, however, owing to drugs, or their pharmacologic dosing, especially cyclophosphamide, which can induce ovarian failure [32]. There are exceptions, however, which are connected to the severity of the disease and to the presence of renal involvement [15].

The impact of pregnancy on SLE activity is variable, and there are contradictory data relating to this issue [9]. This is especially true regarding the effect of pregnancy on the severity of lupus nephritis [75, 76]. It should be noted that evaluating a pregnant patient for the presence of lupus is not simple [9]. For example, certain physiologic changes of pregnancy, such as myalgia; facial, hand, and leg edema; palmar and malar erythema; and changes in hair can imitate SLE [75]. In addition, the serologic expression of SLE may be adversely altered by pregnancy [9]. Antinuclear antibody and proteinuria can be present during pregnancy, without other features of lupus, and preeclamptic toxemia can be difficult to distinguish from lupus nephritis [75]. There is also no clear definition of what constitutes a lupus flare [75], and only very few studies have used standardized measures that have been adapted for use in pregnancy [20].

Older reports, dating from the 1970s or earlier, usually reflected considerable pessimism, with high rates of maternal and fetal complications [76]. In those reports, the exacerbation of SLE was found to vary with the activity of the disease prior to the onset

A. Ingber, *Obstetric Dermatology*,
DOI: 10.1007/978-3-540-88399-9, © Springer-Verlag Berlin Heidelberg 2009

of pregnancy, and tended to be most pronounced during the first 20 weeks of gestation, during delivery, and for several weeks following delivery [24]. In those reports, frequent exacerbations of lupus nephritis had led to 50–82% maternal mortality [76].

Recent reviews of SLE in pregnancy, however, have concluded that the outcome is more favorable than previously thought [23, 38, 64]. A suggested explanation for this difference might stem from the fact that in the past many patients stopped all their therapy when they discovered that they were pregnant. This may well have contributed to the increased risk of disease activation during pregnancy, especially in patients with a history of renal involvement and other forms of serious lupus disease [20].

If we are to summarize all the recent available data, we may rely on several recent studies which have shown a higher rate of flare in lupus patients during pregnancy and 3 months postpartum than in nonpregnant lupus patients during a comparable 12-month period. Most of these flares were mild and responded to low-dose steroids, hydroxychloroquine and/or azathioprine [33, 48, 53].

If SLE first appears during pregnancy it may lead to a higher frequency of severe manifestations, including renal disease, heart failure, fever, lymphadenopathy, abdominal pain with jaundice, and pancreatitis, but even in this group postpartum remission takes place in more than two thirds of cases [23].

Pregnancy was best tolerated by mothers in remission for at least 3 months before conception [1, 13, 38, 64]. Several more recent studies extended this period of time, and reported that the outcome is optimal when the disease is in complete clinical remission for 6–12 months [48, 70]. This is also true for women in remission before pregnancy even with the presence of severe histopathologic changes and heavy proteinuria in the early stages of their disease [23, 28]. Patients with a history of renal involvement are more likely to deteriorate in pregnancy than nonrenal patients. It should be stressed that differentiating active lupus nephritis from preeclampsia is very important, although the two may coexist [20]. In general, if all possible abnormalities are presumed to be due to SLE, disease exacerbation occurs in approximately 25% of patients [38]. If only SLE-specific abnormalities are considered, disease exacerbations occur in 13% of patients [38].

During the active phase of SLE, conception may result in approximately 50% of patients becoming worse during pregnancy. A few will die or experience permanent renal damage; however, this rate of exacerbation may not differ from the rate in nonpregnant women with similar disease severity. To be precise, the flares these patients experience may mirror only the normal course of the disease rather than an influence of pregnancy [75]. It is interesting to see that patients with moderate renal dysfunction (creatinine clearance less than 50 mL/min and proteinuria levels greater than 3 g/day) rarely become pregnant, whereas those with mild dysfunction experience an exacerbation during pregnancy in less than 10% of cases [1]. This may reflect a natural selection that helps to limit the most severe problems [75].

Although older reports have indicated that spontaneous or therapeutic abortion might unfavorably affect maternal SLE [76], a big 1981 study showed no deleterious effects from 15 first-trimester abortions [1].

In relation to the skin, chronic cutaneous lupus is usually considered not to be affected by pregnancy [78]; however, the most common manifestations of SLE in pregnancy are cutaneous flares, followed by arthritis [71]. Common cutaneous manifestations in SLE flares include oral/nasal ulcerations, alopecia, Raynaud's phenomenon, photosensitive skin rash, discoid lupus, malar rash, and subacute cutaneous lupus rash [14]. However, the most common skin lesions seen are painful vasculitic lesions on the extremities [71].

Past reports suggested high incidence of adverse fetal complications in pregnant patients with SLE. Stillbirths, poor head growth, and intrauterine growth retardation have been reported [1, 76]. The rate of spontaneous abortions, especially during the eighth to 14th weeks of gestation, was reported to be 2–4 times the normal rate, and premature birth, with its associated sequelae, was reported to occur in 16–37% of pregnancies after the diagnosis of SLE [24, 64]. However, with optimization of preconceptional diagnostics, pregnancy monitoring, and prophylactic/therapeutic actions, higher rates of live and healthy births in SLE were reported, ranging from 66 to 85% [12, 43]. The effects of SLE on fetal outcome are generally relative to the severity of maternal disease; however, poor fetal outcome may be seen in patients with mild forms of lupus and in whom remission was present at the onset of pregnancy [29, 75].

Transplacental transfer of antinuclear factor may happen, but is not usually detectable in the infant after the age of 6–16 weeks [5, 40]. The infant usually shows no clinical evidence of lupus erythematosus, but rare instances of congenital discoid lupus erythematosus have occurred [39].

Neonatal lupus syndrome is a rare syndrome seen in babies of mothers, most often with circulating anti-Ro (SS-A) antibodies, and can lead to congenital heart block and liver and/or hematologic abnormalities [36, 74]. The most typical feature of neonatal lupus syndrome, however, is a photosensitive rash on the face and scalp. This rash is usually erythematous and scaly but sometimes annular or elliptical, and is often precipitated by exposure to sunlight in the first couple of months after delivery or following UV light treatment for neonatal jaundice. Purpura caused by thrombocytopenia or hemolytic anemia may accompany this condition [69]. The condition is usually self-limiting and necessitates no specific therapy except avoidance of sun exposure for up to 8 months in most cases. For severe rashes, nonfluorinated topical steroids may be used [69].

The antiphospholipid antibody syndrome (APS) presents with thrombosis, recurrent miscarriage, livedo reticularis, migraine, stroke, and/or thrombocytopenia [17, 20]. No formal epidemiologic studies on the incidence of APS in relation to pregnancy have been conducted; however, many investigators in the field feel that patients often present with their first thrombosis in pregnancy or in the first 6 weeks of the postpartum period [20]. Patients with a history of thrombosis must be anticoagulated with low molecular weight heparin in pregnancy, but the optimal dosing regimen is controversial, as is the course of therapy for patients with thromboembolism in pregnancy [7, 18]. APS predisposes to preeclampsia, which may sometimes dictate delivery of the fetus to prevent eclampsia [20].

Management of lupus in pregnancy is complicated by the effects of pregnancy on many of the serologic tests that are used to follow disease activity [75]. Antinuclear antibody, anti-double-stranded deoxyribonucleic acid, and erythrocyte sedimentation rate values have been found to be of limited use [13], and complement levels may not correlate with disease activity [64].

Pharmacologic management of the pregnant patient with SLE requires little modification [1]. In general, corticosteroids are considered reasonably safe for use during pregnancy in careful dosages for appropriate indications [75]. However, steroids should be kept at the minimum dose required to control active lupus as they are associated with an increased risk of pregnancy-induced hypertension, preeclampsia, gestational diabetes, infection, and possible premature rupture of membranes, particularly at dosages above 10 mg daily [48]. In addition, corticosteroids given to laboratory animals during pregnancy have been associated with cleft palate in the offspring, but no such effect has been proved in human beings [1]. These drugs may cause adrenal suppression, and to ensure a proper evaluation of the neonate, the pediatrician should be aware of fetal exposure [35]. Methyl-prednisolone pulses may be given to reduce disease activity quickly in severe cases [48], and there is evidence that increasing the dosage of corticosteroids during labor and in the postpartum period reduces the incidence of postpartum flares of maternal disease [1].

In the case of severe manifestations, such as vasculitis, nephritis, and neuropsychiatric involvement, which could require prolonged high-dose steroid therapy with consequent complications, prednisolone may be replaced with azathiaprine, which is well tolerated, and has not been associated with severe fetal effects, probably because of its degradation by the placenta [41, 76]. Certain drugs such as cyclophosphamide and chlorambucil are highly teratogenic [75].

The use of hemodialysis during pregnancy offers a difficult but suitable means of managing those patients with severe renal disease from many causes and results in a viable though premature or small infant in most cases [1]. Although first-trimester abortions are well tolerated, abortion as a therapeutic modality has been largely abandoned because there is no proved effect on the course of disease [75].

8.2
Systemic Sclerosis

It is not well established whether pregnancy affects systemic sclerosis. The fact that there may be decreased fertility in women with progressive systemic sclerosis, accounting for the low incidence of pregnancy observed in these patients [37], in addition to the fact that many reviews of these subjects were written before 1970 [4, 30, 37, 57], adds to the limited data available. In addition, since the 1970s marked improvement in the prognosis and management of progressive systemic sclerosis has occurred [75].

In the past, studies suggested that immunobiological alterations occurring during pregnancy and the presence of fetal chimeric cells in the mother's tissues might consequently lead to systemic sclerosis and influence the pattern of disease through a disease process similar to graft-versus-host disease. However, there are accumulating up-to-date data suggesting that this phenomenon of perseverance of fetal cells in the mother after pregnancy, also known as microchimerism, is not limited to patients with systemic sclerosis and can be also found in healthy individuals [3, 47]. Accordingly, an Italian case-control study showed that pregnancy does not appear to be a risk factor for the development of systemic sclerosis. There is actually a reduced risk of systemic sclerosis in parous women compared with nulliparous women (age-adjusted odds ratio 0.3; 95% confidence interval 0.1–0.8) [49].

In general, the course of the disease was reported not to be greatly influenced by pregnancy [75]. Slate and Graham [57], who reviewed the records of 66 female patients with scleroderma seen at the Los Angeles County Hospital from January 1951 to July 1964, found that out of 45 of these patients who became pregnant six developed generalized disease during pregnancy. They also found that the average age of death was lower in those patients who had become pregnant than in those who never became pregnant. A more recent study conducted by Steen et al. [61] reported that renal crisis developed in only 17% of 23 women (two during pregnancy) with diffuse cutaneous scleroderma who had one or more pregnancies, which was not statistically different from 22% of 116 patients who were not pregnant during the course of disease. In addition, these same authors found no increased frequency of preeclampsia/eclampsia or hypertension in scleroderma pregnancies [61]. Another study reported a variable effect, with 39% of patients experiencing some worsening of symptoms, whereas 22% noted improvement [30]. It was found that the degree of diffuse skin disease and systemic involvement, particularly lung, cardiac, and renal, are probably more important than the duration of the disease. Limited disease was found to carry a better prognosis for the mother and fetus [9].

The cutaneous manifestations of systemic sclerosis may be categorized into three successive phases [11]. The first phase, the edematous phase, is characterized by complaints of tight, puffy fingers, with nonpitting edema. Later, this phase may be replaced by the indurative phase, characterized by tight, thickened skin, which gradually becomes shiny, taut, and tightly adherent to the subcutis. Color changes frequently occur, with hyperpigmentation and hypopigmentation the most common ones. The last phase – the atrophic phase – demonstrates atrophy of the skin, and the skin becomes thinner than usual. Patients commonly suffer from skin ulcerations and from Raynaud's phenomenon. In relation to these skin manifestations, there are reports that cutaneous sclerosis improved in some persons [4], but worsening sclerodermatous skin change in the postnatal period is not unusual in diffuse systemic sclerosis [58]. Raynaud's phenomenon usually improves during pregnancy, particularly with the increased cardiac output in the second half of pregnancy. Severe cases of Raynaud's phenomenon in pregnancy may be treated with nifedipine, but vasodilators may be discontinued if there is no history of hypertension [58].

Specific effects of pregnancy on two forms of systemic sclerosis – the CREST syndrome (calcinosis, Raynaud's phenomenon, esophageal involvement, sclerodactyly and skin changes in the fingers, telangiectasia) and acrosclerosis – have not been reported.

Although pregnancy usually does not affect scleroderma, exceptions may occur, especially in women suffering from renal disease [76]. Unfortunately, it might be a challenge to detect kidney involvement by regular clinical means at the onset of pregnancy, so it may be impossible to predict which patients will develop complications [76]. Karlen and Cook [31] in a 1974 review reported that pregnancy is usually uneventful until the third trimester, when preeclampsia, hypertension, and renal failure quickly develop, leading to maternal death in all reported cases. They recommended immediate abortion at the first sign of preeclampsia if there is any evidence of deteriorating renal functions [31].

Renal crisis is most common in patients with early diffuse disease, within 5 years of symptom onset [59], and can present before the skin changes, although this is rare [42]. Angiotensin-converting-enzyme inhibitors are considered crucial to control hypertension and the associated renal crisis in pregnant systemic sclerosis patients [8, 59]. This is despite the fact that they are normally not advised in pregnancy, as they have been associated with congenital abnormalities, including infant kidney dysfunction. In contrast to preeclampsia, delivering the fetus does not affect the hypertension or renal dysfunction in such cases [8, 59].

Today, with careful management, a history of renal crisis is not a contraindication to future pregnancy as long as the disease has been stable for several years prior to pregnancy [20].

Systemic sclerosis has historically been associated with fetal loss before and after the onset of disease [6, 54, 56]. A prospective study by Steen [59] published in 1999 reported 91 sclerodermic pregnancies, with a birth rate of 73%, and spontaneous abortion risk of 42% for the subgroup of patients suffering for more than 4 years. Thus, according to recent data and with modern management, fetal loss is similar to that in retrospective controls or first pregnancies except for being increased in late diffuse systemic sclerosis patients [20]. The main problem of pregnant sclerodermic patients is the high risk of preterm delivery, which is reported to have an incidence of 65% for patients afflicted by the systemic type and 23% for others, compared with 5% in controls [20, 59].

Although intrauterine growth retardation has been reported in the pregnancies of women with progressive systemic sclerosis, the true incidence of this event was not established [75], and in a recent large prospective study no small-for-dates babies were born at term [60].

8.3
Dermatomyositis/Polymyositis

There are only a few reports regarding the effect of pregnancy on the course of dermatomyositis/polymyositis (DM/PM). Most of the time the disease is unaffected by pregnancy; however, when it is affected, accumulated data support an agreement that the disease is disadvantageous to both mother and fetus [75]. Remission was noted in only a small percentage of cases [76]. Even with a history of previous normal pregnancies, DM/PM may occur for the first time during gestation, thus demonstrating the ailing effects of pregnancy on this disease [22, 34]. A flare of the heliotrope facial rash and/or proximal muscle weakness was reported to occur in 50% of affected patients [22].

Fetal loss because of abortion, stillbirth, or neonatal death is excessive (46%), and progesterone may aggravate the disease [22, 68]. Unlike the babies of patients with SLE who may suffer from neonatal lupus syndrome, surviving offspring of patients with DM/PM are not affected by the disease [34].

A better prognosis for a successful pregnancy may be achieved with control of the disease [34]. Prednisone, administered in minimal effective doses, is the mainstay of treatment for DM/PM [75]. Cytotoxic drugs generally have not been required [75].

8.4
Pemphigus

Pemphigus vulgaris (PV) is an intraepidermal, immunobullous disease affecting mucous membranes and skin [67]. It is most common in the fifth and the sixth decade [67]. The lesions of pemphigus are flaccid bullae resulting in erosions that heal without scarring [67]. It is caused by an autoantibody directed against the transmembrane components of the desmosome desmogleins 1 and 3 [2]. Direct immunofluorescence studies show an intercellular pattern from the deposition of IgG and C3 in the epidermis. Indirect immunofluorescence tests are positive as well, and there is a good correlation between antibody titers and disease activity [2]. PV is characterized histologically by suprabasilar acantholysis with preserved basal cell dermal adherence [21].

In general, the incidence of PV seems to be coincidental and the course of the disease independent of pregnancy [76], and it is rarely seen in pregnancy [67]. However, PV may occur in pregnancy for the first time or may be aggravated during pregnancy, especially in the first or the second trimester [19, 27] (Figs. 8.1, 8.2). The relative improvement or stabilization of disease during the third trimester has been attributed to the production of endogenous corticosteroids by the placenta in the later stages of pregnancy [46]. The disease can also be provoked by the use of oral contraceptives [27]. The importance of hormones in aggravating the disease was further supported by Honeyman et al. [27], who reported that injection of progesterone intradermally caused acantholytic blisters with deposition of IgG and C3 in the intercellular substance of the epidermis at the site of the injection. This test was administered during a period when the disease was inactive.

In most cases the disease continues in a chronic trend postpartum, although clearing between pregnancies has been observed [75]. It should be emphasized that only a full

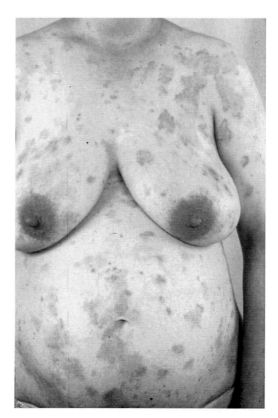

Fig. 8.1 Pemphigus erythematosus. Widespread erosions on an erythemic background in a pregnant woman. The disease appeared at the end of the first trimester

Fig. 8.2 Pemphigus erythematosus.
The same woman as in Fig. 8.1. Typical
lesions on the back

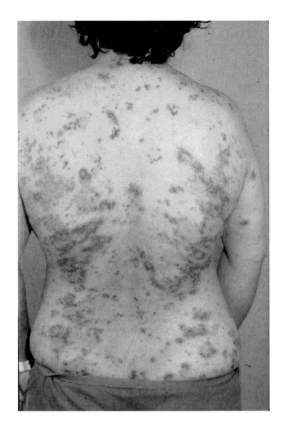

evaluation with skin biopsy and immunofluorescence studies can correctly make the distinction between PV and herpes gestationis because of the similarity in clinical presentation of these two diseases [75].

Transplacental transfer of IgG antibodies may lead to neonatal involvement [21, 44, 65]. Unlike the primary disease, in neonatal disease there is not always a good correlation between antibody titer and disease severity [52]. Neonatal pemphigus has not been reported to progress to primary, adult disease [10], and in afflicted infants the skin cleared and antibodies disappeared from the circulation within 2–3 weeks, with no adverse sequelae [44, 62]. There does not seem to be a direct relationship between the severity of maternal disease and the extent of neonatal involvement [67]. Neonates with extensive disease have been born to women in remission [66], and, conversely, women with active pemphigus have delivered disease-free babies [25, 46, 52]. Because a review of the literature by Ross et al. [51] showed that four of 29 reported cases of pemphigus in pregnancy resulted in stillbirth, the fetus should be considered at risk [75]. Stillborn infants of mothers with pemphigus have been found to have skin lesions and positive direct and indirect immunofluorescence tests characteristic to the disease [21, 65, 73]. However, since recent reports described pemphigus skin lesions and positive immunofluorescence tests also in live births [44, 62], the cause of fetal death cannot be specifically related to pemphigus.

It may be related to maternal drug ingestion (dapsone or prednisone), intercurrent infection, or placental insufficiency [75]. The likelihood of recurrence in following pregnancies is unknown [46].

Pemphigus foliaceous (PF) is characterized by cutaneous involvement and is notable for the absence of oral lesions. Histologically, the epidermal vesicles are located beneath the stratum corneum, in contrast to PV [26].

At least 18 reports of babies born to mothers suffering from PF showed that all of the infants were born free of disease [16, 50]. Only two reports described cases of neonatal PF [26, 72]. Many theories have been suggested to explain the lack of clinical disease in the infants born to mothers with PF. Earlier theories suggested the insignificant titers of PF autoantibodies in the fetal circulation or the lack of reactive antigens on the fetal epidermis may be responsible for this difference [26]. Other theories hypothesized that the placenta, by its barrier function, limits the passage of PF autoantibodies to the baby, or that the placenta serves as an immunoadsorbant of undesirable autoantibodies as suggested by Swinburne [63]. Other explanations may be related to the different allocation of desmogleins in the neonate's epidermis relative to the adult. In neonates desmoglein 3 is expressed in the superficial epidermis, thus providing protection against the formation of blisters induced by PF antibodies [77].

The relation between IgA pemphigus and paraneoplastic pemphigus has not been reported.

Pemphigus during pregnancy is usually treated with high doses of prednisone. Dosages greater than 160 mg daily may be required for initial control, with tapering afterward [21, 44]. Another approach suggests that topical corticosteroids, and only then oral, should be considered as first-line therapy [67]. Azathioprine has been used adjunctively [73], although concerns about the fetal safety of this drug have been expressed [38]. More recently, plasmapheresis has been shown to be useful [55].

Summary

> There is no agreement regarding the effects of pregnancy on the clinical manifestations of *systemic lupus erythematosus* (SLE). Older reports were pessimistic, but recent reviews concluded that the outcome is more favorable. Generally, there is probably a higher rate of flares during pregnancy and 3 months postpartum, but most of them are mild. Pregnancy is best tolerated by mothers in remission for 6–12 months. Management is best achieved by corticosteroids, but azathioprine may be used in severe cases.

> *Chronic cutaneous lupus* is usually considered not to be affected by pregnancy, but the most common manifestations of SLE in pregnancy are cutaneous flares, followed by arthritis.

> *Neonatal lupus syndrome* is a rare syndrome seen in babies of mothers with circulating anti-Ro (SS-A) antibodies, and can lead to congenital heart block, liver and/or hematologic abnormalities. The most typical feature of neonatal lupus syndrome, however, is a photosensitive rash on the face and scalp. The *antiphospholipid antibody syndrome* presents with thrombosis, recurrent miscarriage, livedo reticularis,

Continued

8

Summary *Continued*

migraine, stroke, and/or thrombocytopenia. Some investigators feel that patients often present with their first thrombosis in pregnancy or in the first 6 weeks of the postpartum period.

> It is not well established whether pregnancy affects *systemic sclerosis*. In general, the course of the disease was reported not to be greatly influenced by pregnancy. The degree of skin and systemic involvement is more important than the duration of the disease. Kidney involvement is a risk factor for adverse maternal and fetal outcome, especially during the third trimester.

> Most of the time *dermatomyositis/polymyositis* is unaffected by pregnancy. When it is affected, it usually worsens. Prednisone, administered in minimal effective doses, is the mainstay of treatment.

> *Pemphigus vulgaris* is rarely seen in pregnancy. It may be aggravated during the first and second trimesters. Neonatal involvement may occur, and the fetuses of mothers with pemphigus vulgaris should be considered at risk. In contrast, babies born to *pemphigus foliaceous* patients rarely suffer from the disease.

References

1. Fine LG, Barnett EV, Danovitch GM et al (1981) Systemic lupus erythematosus in pregnancy. Ann Intern Med 94:667–677
2. Anhalt GJ (1999) Making sense of antigens and antibodies in pemphigus. J Am Acad Dermatol 40:763–766
3. Artlett CM (2003) Microchimerism and scleroderma: an update. Curr Rheumatol Rep 5:154–159
4. Ballou SP, Morley JJ, Kushner I (1984) Pregnancy and systemic sclerosis. Arthritis Rheum 27:295–298
5. Beck JS, Oakley CL, Rowell NR (1966) Transplacental passage of antinuclear antibody. Study in infants of mothers with systemic lupus erythematosus. Arch Dermatol 93:656–663
6. Black CM, Stevens WM (1989) Scleroderma. Rheum Dis Clin North Am 15:193–212
7. Branch DW, Khamashta MA (2003) Antiphospholipid syndrome: obstetric diagnosis, management, and controversies. Obstet Gynecol 101:1333–1344
8. Brown AN, Bolster MB (2003) Scleroderma renal crisis in pregnancy associated with massive proteinuria. Clin Exp Rheumatol 21:114–116
9. Buyon JP (1998) The effects of pregnancy on autoimmune diseases. J Leukoc Biol 63:281–287
10. Chowdhury MM, Natarajan S (1998) Neonatal pemphigus vulgaris associated with mild oral pemphigus vulgaris in the mother during pregnancy. Br J Dermatol 139:500–503
11. Chung L, Lin J, Furst DE et al (2006) Systemic and localized scleroderma. Clin Dermatol 24:374–392
12. Clowse ME, Magder LS, Witter F et al (2005) The impact of increased lupus activity on obstetric outcomes. Arthritis Rheum 52:514–521
13. Devoe LD, Taylor RL (1979) Systemic lupus erythematosus in pregnancy. Am J Obstet Gynecol 135:473–479

14. Dhar JP, Sokol RJ (2006) Lupus and pregnancy: complex yet manageable. Clin Med Res 4:310–321
15. Eudy SF, Baker GF (1990) Dermatopathology for the obstetrician. Clin Obstet Gynecol 33:728–737
16. Eyre RW, Stanley JR (1988) Maternal pemphigus foliaceus with cell surface antibody bound in neonatal epidermis. Arch Dermatol 124:25–27
17. Frances C, Piette JC (1997) Cutaneous manifestations of Hughes syndrome occurring in the context of lupus erythematosus. Lupus 6:139–144
18. Ginsberg JS, Bates SM (2003) Management of venous thromboembolism during pregnancy. J Thromb Haemost 1:1435–1442
19. Goldberg NS, DeFeo C, Kirshenbaum N (1993) Pemphigus vulgaris and pregnancy: risk factors and recommendations. J Am Acad Dermatol 28:877–879
20. Gordon C (2004) Pregnancy and autoimmune diseases. Best Pract Res Clin Rheumatol 18:359–379
21. Green D, Maize JC (1982) Maternal pemphigus vulgaris with in vivo bound antibodies in the stillborn fetus. J Am Acad Dermatol 7:388–392
22. Gutierrez G, Dagnino R, Mintz G (1984) Polymyositis/dermatomyositis and pregnancy. Arthritis Rheum 27:291–294
23. Hayslett JP, Reece EA (1985) Systemic lupus erythematosus in pregnancy. Clin Perinatol 12:539–550
24. Hellreich P (1974) The skin changes of pregnancy. Cutis 13:82–86
25. Hern S, Vaughan Jones SA, Setterfield J et al (1998) Pemphigus vulgaris in pregnancy with favourable foetal prognosis. Clin Exp Dermatol 23:260–263
26. Hirsch R, Anderson J, Weinberg JM et al (2003) Neonatal pemphigus foliaceus. J Am Acad Dermatol 49:S187–189
27. Honeyman JF, Eguiguren G, Pinto A et al (1981) Bullous dermatoses of pregnancy. Arch Dermatol 117:264–267
28. Imbasciati E, Surian M, Bottino S et al (1984) Lupus nephropathy and pregnancy. A study of 26 pregnancies in patients with systemic lupus erythematosus and nephritis. Nephron 36:46–51
29. Johnson MJ, Petri M, Witter FR et al (1995) Evaluation of preterm delivery in a systemic lupus erythematosus pregnancy clinic. Obstet Gynecol 86:396–399
30. Johnson TR, Banner EA, Winkelmann RK (1964) Scleroderma and pregnancy. Obstet Gynecol 23:467–469
31. Karlen JR, Cook WA (1974) Renal scleroderma and pregnancy. Obstet Gynecol 44:349–354
32. Khamashta MA, Hughes GR (1996) Pregnancy in systemic lupus erythematosus. Curr Opin Rheumatol 8:424–429
33. Khamashta MA, Ruiz-Irastorza G, Hughes GR (1997) Systemic lupus erythematosus flares during pregnancy. Rheum Dis Clin North Am 23:15–30
34. King CR, Chow S (1985) Dermatomyositis and pregnancy. Obstet Gynecol 66:589–592
35. Lavery JP (1981) Teratology for the dermatologist. Int J Dermatol 20:272–274
36. Lee LA, Lillis PJ, Fritz KA et al (1983) Neonatal lupus syndrome in successive pregnancies. J Am Acad Dermatol 9:401–406
37. Leinwand I, Duryee AW, Richter MN (1954) Scleroderma; based on a study of over 150 cases. Ann Intern Med 41:1003–1041
38. Lockshin MD (1985) Lupus pregnancy. Clin Rheum Dis 11:611–632
39. McCuiston C, Schoch E (1954) Possible discoid lupus erythematosus in a newborn infant: Report of a case with subsequent development of acute systemic lupus erythematosus in mother. Arch Dermatol 70:782–785
40. McKenzie AW (1971) Skin disorders in pregnancy. Practitioner 206:773–780

41. Mecacci F, Pieralli A, Bianchi B et al (2007) The impact of autoimmune disorders and adverse pregnancy outcome. Semin Perinatol 31:223–226

42. Mok CC, Kwan TH, Chow L (2003) Scleroderma renal crisis sine scleroderma during pregnancy. Scand J Rheumatol 32:55–57

43. Molad Y, Borkowski T, Monselise A et al (2005) Maternal and fetal outcome of lupus pregnancy: a prospective study of 29 pregnancies. Lupus 14:145–151

44. Moncada B, Kettelsen S, Hernandez-Moctezuma JL et al (1982) Neonatal pemphigus vulgaris: role of passively transferred pemphigus antibodies. Br J Dermatol 106:465–467

45. Mor-Yosef S, Navot D, Rabinowitz R et al (1984) Collagen diseases in pregnancy. Obstet Gynecol Surv 39:67–84

46. Muhammad JK, Lewis MA, Crean SJ (2002) Oral pemphigus vulgaris occurring during pregnancy. J Oral Pathol Med 31:121–124

47. Nelson JL (2003) Microchimerism in human health and disease. Autoimmunity 36:5–9

48. Petri M (1998) Pregnancy in SLE. Baillieres Clin Rheumatol 12:449–476

49. Pisa FE, Bovenzi M, Romeo L et al (2002) Reproductive factors and the risk of scleroderma: an Italian case-control study. Arthritis Rheum 46:451–456

50. Rocha-Alvarez R, Friedman H, Campbell IT et al (1992) Pregnant women with endemic pemphigus foliaceus (fogo selvagem) give birth to disease-free babies. J Invest Dermatol 99:78–82

51. Ross MG, Kane B, Frieder R et al (1986) Pemphigus in pregnancy: a reevaluation of fetal risk. Am J Obstet Gynecol 155:30–33

52. Ruach M, Ohel G, Rahav D et al (1995) Pemphigus vulgaris and pregnancy. Obstet Gynecol Surv 50:755–760

53. Ruiz-Irastorza G, Lima F, Alves J et al (1996) Increased rate of lupus flare during pregnancy and the puerperium: a prospective study of 78 pregnancies. Br J Rheumatol 35:133–138

54. Scarpinato L, Mackenzie AH (1985) Pregnancy and progressive systemic sclerosis. Case report and review of the literature. Cleve Clin Q 52:207–211

55. Shieh S, Fang YV, Becker JL et al (2004) Pemphigus, pregnancy, and plasmapheresis. Cutis 73:327–329

56. Silman AJ, Black C (1988) Increased incidence of spontaneous abortion and infertility in women with scleroderma before disease onset: a controlled study. Ann Rheum Dis 47:441–444

57. Slate WG, Graham AR (1968) Scleroderma and pregnancy. Am J Obstet Gynecol 101:335–341

58. Steen VD (1997) Scleroderma and pregnancy. Rheum Dis Clin North Am 23:133–147

59. Steen VD (1999) Pregnancy in women with systemic sclerosis. Obstet Gynecol 94:15–20

60. Steen VD, Medsger TA Jr (1999) Fertility and pregnancy outcome in women with systemic sclerosis. Arthritis Rheum 42:763–768

61. Steen VD, Conte C, Day N et al (1989) Pregnancy in women with systemic sclerosis. Arthritis Rheum 32:151–157

62. Storer JS, Galen WK, Nesbitt LT Jr et al (1982) Neonatal pemphigus vulgaris. J Am Acad Dermatol 6:929–932

63. Swinburne LM (1970) Leucocyte antigens and placental sponge. Lancet 2:592–594

64. Syrop CH, Varner MW (1983) Systemic lupus erythematosus. Clin Obstet Gynecol 26:547–557

65. Terpstra H, de Jong MC, Klokke AH (1979) In vivo bound pemphigus antibodies in a stillborn infant. Passive intrauterine transfer of pemphigus vulgaris? Arch Dermatol 115:316–319

66. Tope WD, Kamino H, Briggaman RA et al (1993) Neonatal pemphigus vulgaris in a child born to a woman in remission. J Am Acad Dermatol 29:480–485

67. Torgerson RR, Marnach ML, Bruce AJ et al (2006) Oral and vulvar changes in pregnancy. Clin Dermatol 24:122–132

68. Tsai A, Lindheimer MD, Lamberg SI (1973) Dermatomyositis complicating pregnancy. Obstet Gynecol 41:570–573

69. Tseng CE, Buyon JP (1997) Neonatal lupus syndromes. Rheum Dis Clin North Am 23:31–54
70. Urowitz MB, Gladman DD, Farewell VT et al (1993) Lupus and pregnancy studies. Arthritis Rheum 36:1392–1397
71. Vaughan Jones SA, Black MM (1999) Pregnancy dermatoses. J Am Acad Dermatol 40:233–241
72. Walker DC, Kolar KA, Hebert AA et al (1995) Neonatal pemphigus foliaceus. Arch Dermatol 131:1308–1311
73. Wasserstrum N, Laros RK Jr (1983) Transplacental transmission of pemphigus. JAMA 249:1480–1482
74. Watson RM, Lane AT, Barnett NK et al (1984) Neonatal lupus erythematosus. A clinical, serological and immunogenetic study with review of the literature. Medicine (Baltimore) 63:362–378
75. Winton GB (1989) Skin diseases aggravated by pregnancy. J Am Acad Dermatol 20:1–13
76. Winton GB, Lewis CW (1982) Dermatoses of pregnancy. J Am Acad Dermatol 6:977–998
77. Wu H, Wang ZH, Yan A et al (2000) Protection against pemphigus foliaceus by desmoglein 3 in neonates. N Engl J Med 343:31–35
78. Yell JA, Burge SM (1993) The effect of hormonal changes on cutaneous disease in lupus erythematosus. Br J Dermatol 129:18–22

Tumors in Pregnancy

9

9.1
Mycosis Fungoides

Vonderheid et al. [82] reported in 1981 a patient with mycosis fungoides (MF) who had a flare of disease in three otherwise uncomplicated pregnancies. The patient was unsuccessfully treated, owing to misdiagnosis of psoriasis, with antipsoriatic treatments. A prolonged remission was achieved only 3 years after her last pregnancy owing to topical mechlorethamine hydrochloride treatment [82]. A second case was presented by Castelo-Branco et al. [14], describing a woman with flare up of MF around the conceptional period. In that case MF did not adversely affect pregnancy outcome and gestation did not worsen the course of the malignancy [14].

A third case was reported by Echols et al. [24] in 2001, describing a woman who had been diagnosed with MF 1 year before she became pregnant. She had an acute exacerbation of MF at the beginning of her third trimester that was successfully treated with PUVA and topical steroids. A few weeks later she had a relapse, which was treated with interferon (IFN)-α with a dramatic improvement. She had premature labor complicated by perinatal asphyxia at 36 weeks of pregnancy. The reason for the neonatal stress was not clear, and the patient's disease, IFN therapy, prematurity, and a combination of these were suggested as optional causes [24].

A recent study evaluated seven women with early-stage MF with a total of nine pregnancies [4]. Pregnancy appeared to have no impact on the course of early MF, and no adverse effect was noted on pregnancy [4]; therefore, the effect of pregnancy on the course of MF is not clear, and more descriptions of this disease during pregnancy are needed.

A. Ingber, *Obstetric Dermatology*,
DOI: 10.1007/978-3-540-88399-9, © Springer-Verlag Berlin Heidelberg 2009

9

9.2
Neurofibromatosis

The number and the size of skin lesions of neurofibromas may increase during pregnancy, and new tumors may appear for the first time [12, 75, 85]. At least a partial regression of these lesions is apparent in most instances postpartum [84]. Occasionally, pregnancy may have serious effects on patients with neurofibromatosis. Such a case was described by Ansari and Nagamani [7] in 1976. Their patient had rapid enlargement of plexiform neurofibromas during the last part of pregnancy, resulting in paresis of the lower extremities [7]. In addition, extensive hemorrhage within the tumors led to a sudden drop in hematocrit level, and the patient developed hypertension. Eventually the pregnancy ended with stillbirth of the fetus [7].

Pregnancy might have deleterious effects on the vascular system of patients with neurofibromatosis [84]. Renal artery rupture was reported, and vessel wall rupture into the pleural cavity has led to massive hemothorax [12, 77]. In most cases these events were due to invasion of neurofibromas into the vessel walls [84].

Hypertension occurs regularly in pregnant patients with this syndrome, and Swapp and Main [75] reported its occurrence in ten out of the 11 cases they studied. The reason for this elevation is not known, but it has been suggested that neurofibromatous changes involving the media and elastic layers lead to relative stenosis of the blood vessels, thus causing blood pressure elevation [84].

Owing to the severe deformity and disability and the autosomal dominant mode of transmission, genetic encoding is obligatory for this disease [84, 85]. The most severely affected patients are recommended an elective therapeutic abortion and tubal sterilization [84, 85].

9.3
Melanocytic Nevi

The effect of pregnancy on melanocytic nevi is unclear, and there are few studies that have specifically dealt with this question [22, 44]. In the past, with reliance on several studies, existing cellular nevi (moles) were considered prone to enlarge or darken during pregnancy, and nevi not previously seen were considered to become evident [17, 47, 85]. In a study of 389 pregnant women, 10.5% reported changes in pigmented lesions [65]. No significant histologic abnormalities were seen, however, when compared with controls. In another study of 86 pregnant women, a change in nevi was reported by one third of patients during pregnancy. A mild degree of atypia was reported by histologic examination, but these changes were considered minor, and insufficient to result in diagnostic confusion [31]. A prospective study of 22 patients using photographs and objective measurements for evaluation did not show any significant change in the size of nevi from the first to the third trimester [55]. It has been suggested that patients may overestimate changes in melanocytic nevi [44].

A prospective study which evaluated 17 pregnant women with dysplastic nevus syndrome showed that the rate of change of nevi during pregnancy was twofold higher than when the subjects were not pregnant [25].

Dermoscopic changes in nevi during pregnancy were evaluated in a recent study of 47 pregnant women [89]. Overall dermoscopic changes were mild. There was progressive lightening of the nevi and a progressive decrease in the prominence and thickness of the pigment network. However, vascular structures increased in number, a finding attributed to the general vascular changes seen in pregnancy, and a higher total dermatoscopic score was observed, with a significant reduction in both after delivery.

In conclusion, the clinical feeling that nevi undergo malignant transformations with greater frequency during pregnancy has not been confirmed [85]. Driscoll and Grant-Kells [22] suggest that in view of the fact that the best data available to date suggest that nevi do not typically change over the course of pregnancy, a changing nevus during pregnancy should undergo biopsy, just as in the nonpregnant patient.

9.4
Malignant Melanoma

Malignant melanoma (MM) is a serious global health problem [28]. The incidence of malignant melanoma has been increasing considerably during the past few decades, at a rate that exceeds that of all other solid tumors [28]. The individual lifetime risk for this tumor is now estimated at about 1% [60]. The increasing incidence goes together with a related decrease in the age of presentation [44]. With a peak incidence in the third and fourth decades of life, MM is concentrated among women in their reproductive years [21], and about 30–35% of all women are of childbearing age at diagnosis [16, 54].

The real incidence of MM during pregnancy is unknown [54]. The estimated incidence is between 0.14 and 2.8 cases per 1,000 deliveries [86]. It is considered one of the leading malignancies associated with pregnancy, suggested to account for about 8% of all cancers diagnosed during gestation [56]. From the registry of the German Dermatological Society, it was found that 1% of female melanoma patients were pregnant and 40% were diagnosed during the premenopausal stage [33].

The effect of pregnancy on MM has been debated for almost 60 years, and was considered unclear for many years [52, 84, 85]. Incidental evidence has led to the feeling that endocrine changes may influence tumor behavior [34], and therefore that gestational hyperestrogenic state may increase the risk of MM [83]. Contributing to this impression are the following [21, 67]:

> › There were reports of pregnant females who displayed a rapidly fatal course, manifestation of multiple primary tumors, malignant transformation of congenital and dysplastic nevi during pregnancy, and regression of metastases after delivery. The case report of Riberti et al. [58] exemplifies the circumstantial evidence for the stimulating effect of pregnancy. They reported a pregnant woman in the early weeks of her fifth pregnancy who reported ulceration, bleeding, and rapid increase in the size of a congenital mole on the right forearm [58]. Directly after a spontaneous

9

abortion in the third month of pregnancy, the mole stopped growing, there was no further bleeding, and the local irritation disappeared [58]. Excision of the mole revealed a Clark's level V MM [58]. Of course, whether these changes were directly connected to pregnancy is a matter of interpretation [21].

> Pregnancy is associated with increased pigmentation, due to the stimulation of melanocytes by increased secretion of melanocyte-secreting-hormones and other growth factors [5]. In addition, pregnant women have increased amounts of melano-cyte-stimulating hormone in blood and urine [29].

> Estrogen-receptor proteins were detected in melanoma, congenital nevi, and dysplas-tic nevi, but regularly not in acquired nevi of nonpregnant normal women [15, 26, 27]. This finding was later debated, as studies using sensitive and more specific immu-nohistochemical techniques have not found estrogen receptors (now recognized as estrogen receptor α) in melanoma [23]. Later, Schmidt et al. [66] found that estrogen receptor β and not estrogen receptor α was the predominant estrogen receptor in all types of benign and malignant melanocytic lesions, and that its expression correlates with the malignant tumor microenvironment. Therefore, they stated that estrogen may have a role in MM and that the use of estrogen compounds or topical or oral antiageing treatments should be considered with caution [66].

This impression led to a vast investment in research, both clinical studies and laboratory work. Unfortunately, many clinical reviews suffer from the weakness of retrospective studies and have been questionable [21]. In addition, most large series of pregnant patients with melanoma before 1983 suffer from incomplete histologic data, particularly with regard to tumor thickness [34, 70, 74]; therefore, it is hard to make comparisons with control groups [84].

9.4.1
Maternal Prognosis

This section gives a short description of the available studies evaluating the effect of preg-nancy on melanoma progression and survival. Several controlled studies have reported a decrease in survival rates for pregnant women compared with nonpregnant controls [37, 41, 70, 79]. In 1951 Pack and Scharnagel [52] reported ten patients diagnosed with MM during pregnancy with unfavorable outcomes, but controls were not employed. A retro-spective study by Shiu et al. [70] reviewed 251 cases of MM in women of childbearing age. They compared nulliparous women and those reporting no activation of melanoma during a previous pregnancy with patients who reported activation or who were treated during pregnancy. Increased incidence of stage II disease was present in pregnant women, with metastases present in regional lymph nodes [70]. When stage II disease was present, both conditions were associated with a substantially reduced 5-year survival [70]. Since truncal lesions and ulcerated lesions were more common in the pregnant group, this outcome was expected. The authors suggested that pregnancy may have an influence on the course of some melanomas and that the effects may be most obvious in those with the greatest risk of residual disease after treatment [70].

Lower survival in pregnant melanoma patients was also reported by Houghton et al. [37]. A 55% 5-year survival rate was reported in 12 patients diagnosed with MM during pregnancy compared with 83% in nonpregnant age-matched controls. These patients also had a propensity to have thicker lesions that were frequently located on the trunk, both poor prognostic signs [37]. After matching for the site and the thickness of primary lesions, they found no difference in prognosis [37].

The only controlled study that shows a decrease in survival rate after matching for age, tumor site, and stage, is a Russian study by Trapeznikov et al. [79] reviewed by Kjems and Krag [41]. This study compared 102 women with melanoma during pregnancy with 599 nonpregnant controls. After 10 years of follow-up, the pregnant group had a 26% survival rate compared with a 43% survival rate in the nonpregnant group, which is a statistically significant difference. As mentioned above, this study matched for all prognostic factors, thus suggesting that the reduced 10-year survival is the result of pregnancy alone.

Other controlled studies show no statistically significant difference in survival rates [46, 48, 57, 73, 86], although some of these studies were limited by the length of follow-up [57, 86]. In addition, although no significant decrease in survival has been reported, some studies showed a significantly shorter disease-free interval (DFI) in pregnant women, possibly ascribed to a shortened time to nodal metastasis [57,72,73].

George et al. [34] compared 115 patients who were pregnant at presentation or had a following pregnancy after treatment with 141 nonpregnant patients of similar ages. The 10-year survival rates of the two groups were about the same, being 42% in the pregnant group and 45% in the nonpregnant group. However, they found that melanomas associated with pregnancy in general were in a more advanced stage at the time of diagnosis and treatment than in those patients who were not pregnant [34]. This difference might be related to different expression of biologic potential or to a delay in diagnosis by the physicians [34].

Shiu et al. [70] found no differences in the 5-year, disease-free survival rates related to pregnancy or activation in patients with stage I melanoma (tumor limited to the primary site with no metastases in regional lymph nodes). They found, however, that pregnant patients had a higher incidence of lesions which bleed, ulcerate, or become elevated [70]. Reintgen et al. [57] studied 58 pregnant patients with melanoma, with comparison of histologic data. Survival rates for patients in whom melanoma developed during pregnancy were the same as in a control group of nonpregnant women with histologically similar tumors. The disease-free interval (DFI), however, was shorter in the pregnant group [57]. This apparent inconsistency may be due to the small number of patients in both groups who died within 5 years, which led to a decreased chance of finding a significant difference in survival [84]. A second group of 46 patients who had become pregnant within 5 years of diagnosis of melanoma was also studied [57], and similarly no differences in survival characteristics were found [57].

McManamny et al. [48] studied 23 pregnant women who were diagnosed with MM during pregnancy. There was no significance in survival or DFI between those patients and controls [48]. Wong et al. [87] found that pregnancy did not affect survival rates of 66 women with melanoma diagnosed during pregnancy. In contrast to the findings of Reintgen et al. [57], the mean DFI was actually longer in the pregnant patients than in controls.

In 1992 Slingluff and Seigler [71] followed 100 patients diagnosed with melanoma during pregnancy for a mean of 6.8 years. On the whole, the mortality rate was 25% for the

9

pregnant group compared with 23% for the nonpregnant group, a difference that was not statistically significant. 48% of pregnant women had nodal metastases in comparison with 26% of the nonpregnant women, and a significantly shorter DFI for the pregnant group was found. It was suggested that if the patients were followed for a longer time this shortened DIF would lead to a lower survival rate for the pregnant population [8].

MacKie et al. [46] studied the effect of pregnancy on the prognosis in 388 women with stage I melanoma before, during, after, and between pregnancies Women who were treated for MM during pregnancy had a worse prognosis and a shorter disease-free survival compared with controls. They also found that head, neck, and truncal lesions were observed in 43% of pregnant patients compared with 38% of nonpregnant controls, $P = 0.009$ [46]. After matching for tumor thickness, they found the differences became statistically insignificant. It should be noted, however, that if pregnancy has a negative effect on the course of MM by inducing the proliferation of cancerous cells, then controlling for tumor thickness would lead to wrong interpretation of the results [2].

Daryanani et al. [18] evaluated 46 pregnant women diagnosed with MM during pregnancy, with generation of 10-year survival and DFI curves. There was no significant difference in survival rate or DFI [18]. A recent retrospective cohort study of 185 melanoma patients diagnosed during pregnancy using data from the Swedish National and Regional Registries showed no statistically significant difference in overall survival between pregnant and nonpregnant groups [43]. Another large case-controlled study using records from the California Cancer Registry compared 289 women with localized, pregnancy-associated MM with 1,716 controls [51]. No significant difference in survival based on 10-year Kaplan–Meier survival curves was found.

In summary, there is some support for the suggestion that pregnancy may be associated with advanced stages of disease, an increase in poor prognostic sites, thicker lesions, a shorter disease-free survival period, and a decrease in 10-year survival rate [8]. However, according to recent clinical trails, there is now strong evidence that the clinical course of pregnant women with melanoma is similar to that of nonpregnant women [54]. There are insufficient data with respect to the effects on stage III and stage IV melanoma [49]. More long-term follow-up is needed to confirm a survival disadvantage [8].

9.4.2
Fetal Prognosis

Transplacental transmission of melanoma to the fetus, with consequent fatal metastasis after parturition, has been reported, and it is the most common cancer to metastasize to the products of conception [19, 52, 62]. It is responsible for 30% of the reported cases of metastasis [8], and for 58% of those cases in which a fetus was involved [13, 19]. The usual case of maternal melanoma, however, has no adverse effect on the fetus [84]. In addition, fetal metastasis occurs in only 25% of cases with metastasis to the conceptus [10]. Therefore, therapeutic abortions for patients with stage I or stage II disease is not indicated [59]. Patients with stage III disease who will undergo adjuvant therapy should consider therapeutic abortions in the first trimester because of unknown effects of the therapy on the fetus [78].

When melanoma occurs during pregnancy, clinical and histologic examination of the placenta is necessary postpartum, since occult, metastatic disease to the fetal liver can occur

[84]. The only evidence of such an event might be placental tumor implantation [52]. If it is present, the infant should be monitored for development of malignant disease, including frequent skin examination by the dermatologist [22, 44]. Of seven reported cases of MM affecting the newborn or fetus, five newborns died of metastatic MM within hours to 11 months after delivery. The others had "spontaneous resolution" of disease [3, 6, 10, 19, 30].

9.4.3
Treatment

Any suspicious change in a pigmented cutaneous lesion during pregnancy deserves a biopsy, and a diagnosis of melanoma should be treated rapidly and sufficiently without compromising the patient's chance for cure [21]. It should be remembered that pregnancy is a secondary concern in potentially curable patients [21].

Treatment of MM relies on wide surgical excision with fitting margins (depending on the thickness of the primary lesion) [80, 81]. Lesions less than 1.0 mm thick should be excised with a 1.0-cm border, whereas intermediate-thickness melanoma (1–4 mm) warrants 2.0-cm margins [59]. This procedure can be carried out under local anesthesia, with little risk to the fetus. Lidocaine is a pregnancy category B drug according to the Food and Drug Administration classification, and is safe for local anesthesia during pregnancy [76]. Epinephrine is classified as a category C drug by the Food and Drug Administration [42], and it has been suggested that it can be used safely in pregnancy if used cautiously [61].

Sentinel lymph node mapping is often recommended for patients with lesions 1–4 mm in size [59], and it has been shown to be accurate with little morbidity and high accuracy [44] Although the blue dye involved does not give rise to ionizing radiation, the technetium present results in insignificant exposure of the fetus ionizing radiation (400 µCi) [59]. Since most of the radiation dose is localized to the injection site or within the lymphatics, it seems that the benefits of sentinel node mapping surpass the risk to the fetus [50]. According to the University of Michigan, the risk of anaphylaxis to isosulfan blue dye is one of the principal safety concerns for pregnant women, and therefore radiocolloid alone is used for sentinel lymph node mapping and biopsy [68]. Another major melanoma center in the UK does not perform sentinel lymph node biopsy and mapping for women under 30 weeks' gestation because of the potential impact on fetal organogenesis, which becomes most critical at the end of the first trimester [45].

If lymph node dissection under general anesthesia is indicated, the surgery should ideally be performed during the second trimester owing to evidence of increased teratogenicity and abortion in the first trimester and increased risk of spontaneous abortion during the third trimester [59].

The performance of radiologic examinations in the pregnant patient should be considered according to the existence of symptoms, the stage of pregnancy, the specific test needed, and the estimated dose of ionizing radiation and the risks associated with that dose. Women with early disease should not undergo intensive radiologic investigation [44]. A posteroanterior and lateral chest radiograph is recommended by the National Institutes of Health in patients with melanoma measuring more than 1.0 mm [59]. According to Nicklas and Baker [50], a chest radiograph result in minor irradiation of fetus, with an estimated dose of 0.6 mGy (or 0.06 mrad), and is not contraindicated in the pregnant patient, especially when used with proper shielding. Shapiro [69] stated that in early pregnancy, sonographic assessment of the abdomen and liver is favored over computed tomographic scanning with intravenous contrast material, because of the absorbed fetal radiation dose. Magnetic resonance imaging is safer than computed tomographic scanning, but it is not suggested during the first trimester because of the heating of tissues connected with the radiofrequency fields used during magnetic resonance imaging [45].

Metastatic disease to lymph nodes and isolated metastases to the lungs, gastrointestinal tract, and brain may be palliated by surgical removal or with chemotherapy, although with limited success [88]. Chemotherapeutic agents used in metastatic melanoma include dacarbazine and combinations such as tamoxifen, carmustine, and cisplatin [20]. Several case reports regarding treatment of metastatic melanoma during pregnancy have been published [16, 73]. Dacarbazine was given for a pregnant patient with MM. Although she gave birth to a healthy male infant and had dramatic remission with therapy, she relapsed and died 8 weeks postpartum [35]. The use of adjuvant IFN-α_{2b} in patients with high-risk melanoma is debatable [39,40]. It has been used safely in several conditions during pregnancy, such as to treat hepatitis, myeloproliferative disorders, and multiple myeloma [9, 63, 64]. However, adjuvant IFN therapy for MM warrants higher doses, which involve major side effects such as influenza-like symptoms [83]. The toxicity of this high-dose IFN therapy in pregnant patients was not studied [83].

Whether women with melanoma should plan future pregnancies or use oral contraceptives is a difficult question [84]. Several studies have compared the use of oral contraceptive pills in melanoma patients with use by control groups of healthy women [1, 11, 32, 36], but only two have found a statistically significantly greater use in patients [11, 36]. Neither of those studies controlled for sun exposure, a much more important factor in the development of melanoma than low-level hormonal factors [84]. In addition, although there are fewer studies, epidemiologic evidence to date has not shown an enhanced risk of MM from use of hormone replacement therapy [22]. Therefore, if a woman who was diagnosed and treated for MM has a need to use either oral contraceptive pills or hormone replacement therapy, and other alternative therapies do not exist, these exogenous hormones are not contraindicated [22].

If reappearance of disease happens, it usually develops in the first 5 years, with 60–70% of diseases developing within the first 2 years and 80–90% within 5 years [59]. On the basis of these data, many practitioners recommend that all women with this disease avoid pregnancy for 2–5 years after treatment if there is no evidence of recurrent malignancy [48, 58, 78, 83]. Women whose melanoma did not occur during pregnancy need not adhere to these guidelines, as their tumor did not show evidence of hormonal stimulation [84]. There is no evidence that a diagnosis of melanoma adversely affects fertility [44].

9.5
Miscellaneous

Anetoderma of Jadassohn (dermatochalasis; macular atrophy) was described by DeOreo in 1951, occurring in a patient during the first month of pregnancy [17]. Atrophic lesions developed on the trunk, arms, and thighs over a 3-month period [17]. This association is rare and perhaps coincidental [85].

One or more dermatofibromas commonly develop during pregnancy [17]. Leiomyomas may double in size or become painful [17]. Keloids may grow rapidly [85]. Cases of accelerated growth of dermatofibrosarcoma protuberans, an uncommon tumor of the dermis, during pregnancy have been reported [53]. This tumor is known to be affected by platelet-derived growth factor and progesterone, thus possibly explaining its rapid growth during gestation [38].

Desmoid tumors are firm, nontender, subcutaneous masses that arise from muscular aponeuroses [85]. They usually develop in the rectus abdominis muscle during pregnancy or following childbirth or trauma [85]. Although they are benign, fibrous neoplasms, they may be locally destructive, and wide, local excision is recommended [85].

Summary

> Although it was thought that melanocytic nevi change in pregnancy and might even undergo malignant transformation, this was not confirmed. A changing nevus during pregnancy should undergo biopsy, just as in the nonpregnant patient.

> Malignant melanoma (MM) is considered one of the leading malignancies associated with pregnancy, and about 30–35% of all women are of childbearing age at diagnosis.

> Pregnancy may have a connection to more advanced stages of disease, thicker lesions, shorter disease-free survival, and reduced 10-year survival rate. However, recent clinical studies suggest that the clinical course is similar to that of nonpregnant women.

> MM is the most common cancer to metastasize to the products of conception, and fetal death due to MM has been reported. Therefore, examination of the placenta is necessary postpartum.

> MM in pregnancy should be treated in the same manner as in the nonpregnant state. Some recommend avoiding pregnancy for 2–5 years after treatment.

> The number and the size of skin lesions of neurofibromas may increase during pregnancy, and new tumors may appear for the first time. Hypertension occurs regularly in pregnant patients with this syndrome.

> There are also reports of adverse effects of pregnancy on the course of mycosis fungoides, dermatofibromas, keloids, leiomyomas, and desmoid tumors.

References

1. Adam SA, Sheaves JK, Wright NH et al (1981) A case-control study of the possible association between oral contraceptives and malignant melanoma. Br J Cancer 44:45–50
2. Adami HO, Thorn M, Bergstrom R et al (1991) Melanoma in pregnancy. Lancet 337:1164–1165
3. Alexander A, Harris RM, Grossman D et al (2004) Vulvar melanoma: diffuse melanosis and metastasis to the placenta. J Am Acad Dermatol 50:293–298

4. Amitay-Layish I, David M, Kafri B et al (2007) Early-stage mycosis fungoides, parapsoriasis en plaque, and pregnancy. Int J Dermatol 46:160–165
5. Ances IG, Pomerantz SH (1974) Serum concentrations of beta-melanocyte-stimulating hormone in human pregnancy. Am J Obstet Gynecol 119:1062–1068
6. Anderson JF, Kent S, Machin GA (1989) Maternal malignant melanoma with placental metastasis: a case report with literature review. Pediatr Pathol 9:35–42
7. Ansari AH, Nagamani M (1976) Pregnancy and neurofibromatosis (von Recklinghausen's disease). Obstet Gynecol 47:25SS–29SS
8. Antonelli NM, Dotters DJ, Katz VL et al (1996) Cancer in pregnancy: a review of the literature. Part I. Obstet Gynecol Surv 51:125–134
9. Baer MR (1991) Normal full-term pregnancy in a patient with chronic myelogenous leukemia treated with alpha-interferon. Am J Hematol 37:66
10. Baergen RN, Johnson D, Moore T et al (1997) Maternal melanoma metastatic to the placenta: a case report and review of the literature. Arch Pathol Lab Med 121:508–511
11. Beral V, Ramcharan S, Faris R (1977) Malignant melanoma and oral contraceptive use among women in California. Br J Cancer 36:804–809
12. Brady DB, Bolan JC (1984) Neurofibromatosis and spontaneous hemothorax in pregnancy: two case reports. Obstet Gynecol 63:35S–38S
13. Brossard J, Abish S, Bernstein ML et al (1994) Maternal malignancy involving the products of conception: a report of malignant melanoma and medulloblastoma. Am J Pediatr Hematol Oncol 16:380–383
14. Castelo-Branco C, Torne A, Cararach V et al (2001) Mycosis fungoides and pregnancy. Oncol Rep 8:197–199
15. Chaudhuri PK, Walker MJ, Briele HA et al (1980) Incidence of estrogen receptor in benign nevi and human malignant melanoma. JAMA 244:791–793
16. Colbourn DS, Nathanson L, Belilos E (1989) Pregnancy and malignant melanoma. Semin Oncol 16:377–387
17. Cummings K, Derbes V (1967) Dermatoses associated with pregnancy. Cutis 3:120–125
18. Daryanani D, Plukker JT, De Hullu JA et al (2003) Pregnancy and early-stage melanoma. Cancer 97:2248–2253
19. Dildy GA 3rd, Moise KJ Jr, Carpenter RJ Jr et al (1989) Maternal malignancy metastatic to the products of conception: a review. Obstet Gynecol Surv 44:535–540
20. Dipaola RS, Goodin S, Ratzell M et al (1997) Chemotherapy for metastatic melanoma during pregnancy. Gynecol Oncol 66:526–530
21. Donegan WL (1983) Cancer and pregnancy. CA Cancer J Clin 33:194–214
22. Driscoll MS, Grant-Kels JM (2007) Hormones, nevi, and melanoma: an approach to the patient. J Am Acad Dermatol 57:919–931; quiz 932–916
23. Duncan LM, Travers RL, Koerner FC et al (1994) Estrogen and progesterone receptor analysis in pregnancy-associated melanoma: absence of immunohistochemically detectable hormone receptors. Hum Pathol 25:36–41
24. Echols KT, Gilles JM, Diro M (2001) Mycosis fungoides in pregnancy: remission after treatment with alpha-interferon in a case refractory to conventional therapy: a case report. J Matern Fetal Med 10:68–70
25. Ellis DL (1991) Pregnancy and sex steroid hormone effects on nevi of patients with the dysplastic nevus syndrome. J Am Acad Dermatol 25:467–482
26. Ellis DL, Wheeland RG, Solomon H (1985) Estrogen and progesterone receptors in congenital melanocytic nevi. J Am Acad Dermatol 12:235–244

27. Ellis DL, Wheeland RG, Solomon H (1985) Estrogen and progesterone receptors in melano-cytic lesions. Occurrence in patients with dysplastic nevus syndrome. Arch Dermatol 121:1282–1285
28. Errickson CV, Matus NR (1994) Skin disorders of pregnancy. Am Fam Physician 49:605–610
29. Eudy SF, Baker GF (1990) Dermatopathology for the obstetrician. Clin Obstet Gynecol 33:728–737
30. Ferreira CM, Maceira JM, Coelho JM (1998) Melanoma and pregnancy with placental metas-tases. Report of a case. Am J Dermatopathol 20:403–407
31. Foucar E, Bentley TJ, Laube DW et al (1985) A histopathologic evaluation of nevocellular nevi in pregnancy. Arch Dermatol 121:350–354
32. Gallagher RP, Elwood JM, Hill GB et al (1985) Reproductive factors, oral contraceptives and risk of malignant melanoma: Western Canada Melanoma Study. Br J Cancer 52:901–907
33. Garbe C (1993) Pregnancy, hormone preparations and malignant melanoma. Hautarzt 44:347–352
34. George PA, Fortner JG, Pack GT (1960) Melanoma with pregnancy. A report of 115 cases. Cancer 13:854–859
35. Harkin KP, Drumm JE, O'Brien P et al (1990) Metastatic malignant melanoma in pregnancy. Ir Med J 83:116–117
36. Holly EA, Weiss NS, Liff JM (1983) Cutaneous melanoma in relation to exogenous hormones and reproductive factors. J Natl Cancer Inst 70:827–831
37. Houghton AN, Flannery J, Viola MV (1981) Malignant melanoma of the skin occurring during pregnancy. Cancer 48:407–410
38. Kikuchi K, Soma Y, Fujimoto M et al (1993) Dermatofibrosarcoma protuberans: increased growth response to platelet-derived growth factor BB in cell culture. Biochem Biophys Res Commun 196:409–415
39. Kirkwood JM (1998) Systemic adjuvant treatment of high-risk melanoma: the role of inter-feron alfa-2b and other immunotherapies. Eur J Cancer 34(Suppl 3):S12–17
40. Kirkwood JM, Strawderman MH, Ernstoff MS et al (1996) Interferon alfa-2b adjuvant therapy of high-risk resected cutaneous melanoma: the Eastern Cooperative Oncology Group Trial EST 1684. J Clin Oncol 14:7–17
41. Kjems E, Krag C (1993) Melanoma and pregnancy. A review. Acta Oncol 32:371–378
42. Lawrence C (1996) Drug management in skin surgery. Drugs 52:805–817
43. Lens MB, Rosdahl I, Ahlbom A et al (2004) Effect of pregnancy on survival in women with cutaneous malignant melanoma. J Clin Oncol 22:4369–4375
44. Lishner M (2003) Cancer in pregnancy. Ann Oncol 14(Suppl 3):iii31–iii36
45. Lloyd MS, Topping A, Allan R et al (2004) Contraindications to sentinel lymph node biopsy in cutaneous malignant melanoma. Br J Plast Surg 57:725–727
46. MacKie RM, Bufalino R, Morabito A et al (1991) Lack of effect of pregnancy on outcome of melanoma. For The World Health Organisation Melanoma Programme. Lancet 337:653–655
47. McKenzie AW (1971) Skin disorders in pregnancy. Practitioner 206:773–780
48. McManamny DS, Moss AL, Pocock PV et al (1989) Melanoma and pregnancy: a long-term follow-up. Br J Obstet Gynaecol 96:1419–1423
49. Muallem MM, Rubeiz NG (2006) Physiological and biological skin changes in pregnancy. Clin Dermatol 24:80–83
50. Nicklas AH, Baker ME (2000) Imaging strategies in the pregnant cancer patient. Semin Oncol 27:623–632
51. O'Meara AT, Cress R, Xing G et al (2005) Malignant melanoma in pregnancy. A population-based evaluation. Cancer 103:1217–1226

52. Pack GT, Scharnagel IM (1951) The prognosis for malignant melanoma in the pregnant woman. Cancer 4:324–334
53. Parlette LE, Smith CK, Germain LM et al (1999) Accelerated growth of dermatofibrosarcoma protuberans during pregnancy. J Am Acad Dermatol 41:778–783
54. Pavlidis NA (2002) Coexistence of pregnancy and malignancy. Oncologist 7:279–287
55. Pennoyer JW, Grin CM, Driscoll MS et al (1997) Changes in size of melanocytic nevi during pregnancy. J Am Acad Dermatol 36:378–382
56. Potter JF, Schoeneman M (1970) Metastasis of maternal cancer to the placenta and fetus. Cancer 25:380–388
57. Reintgen DS, McCarty KS, Jr, Vollmer R et al (1985) Malignant melanoma and pregnancy. Cancer 55:1340–1344
58. Riberti C, Marola G, Bertani A (1981) Malignant melanoma: the adverse effect of pregnancy. Br J Plast Surg 34:338–339
59. Richards KA, Stasko T (2002) Dermatologic surgery and the pregnant patient. Dermatol Surg 28:248–256
60. Rigel DS, Kopf AW, Friedman RJ (1987) The rate of malignant melanoma in the United States: are we making an impact? J Am Acad Dermatol 17:1050–1053
61. Rosenberg PH, Veering BT, Urmey WF (2004) Maximum recommended doses of local anesthetics: a multifactorial concept. Reg Anesth Pain Med 29:564–575; discussion 524
62. Rothman LA, Cohen CJ, Astarloa J (1973) Placental and fetal involvement by maternal malignancy: a report of rectal carcinoma and review of the literature. Am J Obstet Gynecol 116:1023–1034
63. Ruggiero G, Andreana A, Zampino R (1996) Normal pregnancy under inadvertent alpha-interferon therapy for chronic hepatitis C. J Hepatol 24:646
64. Sakata H, Karamitsos J, Kundaria B et al (1995) Case report of interferon alfa therapy for multiple myeloma during pregnancy. Am J Obstet Gynecol 172:217–219
65. Sanchez JL, Figueroa LD, Rodriguez E (1984) Behavior of melanocytic nevi during pregnancy. Am J Dermatopathol 6(Suppl):89–91
66. Schmidt AN, Nanney LB, Boyd AS et al (2006) Oestrogen receptor-beta expression in melanocytic lesions. Exp Dermatol 15:971–980
67. Schwartz BK, Zashin SJ, Spencer SK et al (1987) Pregnancy and hormonal influences on malignant melanoma. J Dermatol Surg Oncol 13:276–281
68. Schwartz JL, Mozurkewich EL, Johnson TM (2003) Current management of patients with melanoma who are pregnant, want to get pregnant, or do not want to get pregnant. Cancer 97:2130–2133
69. Shapiro RL (2002) Surgical approaches to malignant melanoma. Practical guidelines. Dermatol Clin 20:681–699, ix
70. Shiu MH, Schottenfeld D, Maclean B et al (1976) Adverse effect of pregnancy on melanoma: a reappraisal. Cancer 37:181–187
71. Slingluff CL Jr, Seigler HF (1992) Malignant melanoma and pregnancy. Ann Plast Surg 28:95–99
72. Slingluff CL Jr, Reintgen D (1993) Malignant melanoma and the prognostic implications of pregnancy, oral contraceptives, and exogenous hormones. Semin Surg Oncol 9:228–231
73. Slingluff CL Jr, Reintgen DS, Vollmer RT et al (1990) Malignant melanoma arising during pregnancy. A study of 100 patients. Ann Surg 211:552–557; discussion 558–559
74. Sutherland CM, Loutfi A, Mather FJ et al (1983) Effect of pregnancy upon malignant melanoma. Surg Gynecol Obstet 157:443–446
75. Swapp GH, Main RA (1973) Neurofibromatosis in pregnancy. Br J Dermatol 88:431–435
76. Sweeney SM, Maloney ME (2006) Pregnancy and dermatologic surgery. Dermatol Clin 24:205–214, vi

77. Tapp E, Hickling RS (1969) Renal artery rupture in a pregnant woman with neurofibromatosis. J Pathol 97:398–402

78. Teplitzky S, Sabates B, Yu K et al (1998) Melanoma during pregnancy: a case report and review of the literature. J La State Med Soc 150:539–543

79. Trapeznikov NN, Khasanov SR, Iavorskii VV (1987) Melanoma of the skin and pregnancy. Vopr Onkol 33:40–46

80. Veronesi U, Cascinelli N (1991) Narrow excision (1-cm margin). A safe procedure for thin cutaneous melanoma. Arch Surg 126:438–441

81. Veronesi U, Cascinelli N, Adamus J et al (1988) Thin stage I primary cutaneous malignant melanoma. Comparison of excision with margins of 1 or 3 cm. N Engl J Med 318:1159–1162

82. Vonderheid EC, Dellatorre DL, Van Scott EJ (1981) Prolonged remission of tumor-stage mycosis fungoides by topical immunotherpay. Arch Dermatol 117:586–589

83. Weisz B, Schiff E, Lishner M (2001) Cancer in pregnancy: maternal and fetal implications. Hum Reprod Update 7:384–393

84. Winton GB (1989) Skin diseases aggravated by pregnancy. J Am Acad Dermatol 20:1–13

85. Winton GB, Lewis CW (1982) Dermatoses of pregnancy. J Am Acad Dermatol 6:977–998

86. Wong DJ, Strassner HT (1990) Melanoma in pregnancy. Clin Obstet Gynecol 33:782–791

87. Wong JH, Sterns EE, Kopald KH et al (1989) Prognostic significance of pregnancy in stage I melanoma. Arch Surg 124:1227–1230; discussion 1230–1221

88. Wornom IL 3rd, Smith JW, Soong SJ et al (1986) Surgery as palliative treatment for distant metastases of melanoma. Ann Surg 204:181–185

89. Zampino MR, Corazza M, Costantino D et al (2006) Are melanocytic nevi influenced by pregnancy? A dermoscopic evaluation. Dermatol Surg 32:1497–1504

Metabolic Diseases in Pregnancy

10

10.1
Porphyria Cutanea Tarda

Waldenstrom [27] first described porphyria cutanea tarda (PCT) in 1937. It is the most common disorder of porphyrin metabolism in Europe and North America [14], with an estimated incidence of one in 70,000 [19]. PCT encompasses a heterogeneous group of disorders – acquired (sporadic or type I) or inherited (familial or type II) as an autosomal dominant trait [1]. Both sporadic and familial PCT are known to be adversely influenced by external factors, of which the most commonly incriminated are estrogen, hepatitis C infection, iron overload, and alcohol intake [14, 20, 28]. Pregnancy and the postpartum period, as well as estrogen-containing birth control pills, have been reported, although scarcely in the literature, to exacerbate this condition [1, 2, 9, 13, 14, 22, 25]. There is only a single report regarding the manifestation of PCT postpartum [15]. Two patients developed mild preeclampsia and one gestational diabetes during the course of their pregnancy [2, 14].

Orally administered estrogens and endogenous estrogens formed during pregnancy probably exert different effects on PCT [21]. There are case reports of PCT patients whose disease was not exacerbated by pregnancy, leading to the speculation that endogenous estrogens may not be harmful or that the effects estrogen on PCT have been overstated [2, 8, 9, 13, 17]. Orally administered estrogens significantly increase the levels of renin substrate, thyroxine-binding globulin, and cortisol-binding globulin, all of which are produced by hepatic metabolism [21]. Endogenous production of estrogens bypasses the first-pass effect in the liver; therefore, oral estrogens, and not estrogens formed during pregnancy, are more likely to provoke the disease [25].

There are, however, several reports that show an obvious deterioration of disease symptomatically and increases in the levels of plasma and urine porphyrins during gestation and in the postpartum period [2, 13, 14, 22]. Usually there is a clinical deterioration during the first trimester, overlapping with a physiologic rise in serum estrogen levels and a high rate of excretion of porphyrins [13]. Later in pregnancy, during the second and third trimesters,

there is a decrease in placental estrogen and progesterone production, fetal iron require-
ments rise and blood volume increases and lead to hemodilution. Therefore, the skin disease improves and an associated fall in the levels of serum iron and urinary porphyrins and
coproporphyrins occurs [13]. The use of medications during pregnancy can also precipitate
or exacerbate the disorder and should be avoided [14]. For example, barbiturates lead to
redirection of heme into synthesis of monooxygenases for their own metabolism, increasing porphyrin precursors [14]. Griseofulvin and rifampicin can induce -aminolevulinic
acid synthetase activity, and worsen the disease [8].

Pregnancy may also be affected by this disease [14]. The liver may be involved in
PCT patients, leading to liver dysfunction and chronic liver disease, which may be
associated with hepatotropic viruses [14]. Unexplained benign elevations in aspartate
aminotransferase and alanine aminotransferase levels that resolve or improve postpartum have been reported during pregnancy [14]. The reason for these elevations has
been suggested to result from limited hemosiderosis, fatty and moderate mononuclear
liver infiltration precipitated by the disorder [14]. Patients with PCT have a high incidence of hepatitis B and C, both by antibody testing and polymerase chain reaction;
therefore, the staff, the mothers, and the newborns should be appropriately protected
and treated [14, 18].

Sixty percent of patients with PCT are at risk for abnormal glucose tolerance and overt
diabetes [13]; therefore, patients should be screened with fasting glucose levels [14].
Thirty-six percent of PCT patients test positive for antinuclear antibody, which may have
important implications for the pregnancy, although it is at present unknown whether these
patients are at increased risk for recurrent pregnancy loss [14]. Nevertheless, it is recommended to test for lupus anticoagulant and anticardiolipin antibodies [14]. A high incidence of preeclampsia has been noted among PCT patients. For that reason, treatment with
low-dose aspirin may be worthwhile for patients who test positive [14]. Because increasing
numbers of acquired immunodeficiency disease cases and PCT have been reported [6],
patients presenting with PCT and risk factors for HIV infection should be tested for HIV
and treated accordingly [3].

Because few cases have been reported in the literature, little is known about their management. In general, the management during pregnancy includes observation and avoidance of alcohol, iron (unless iron deficiency anemia is demonstrable), and exposure to
sunlight, especially during the first trimester, because the clinical manifestations of PCT
improve as the pregnancy advances [1, 14]. In patients with multiple recurrences or those
who do not show signs of improvement by the second trimester, the use of repeated phlebotomies, with careful monitoring of hematocrit levels, has been used successfully in the
past to reduce the red blood cell volume and decrease porphyrin excretion. Phlebotomy
consists of venesection twice weekly of about 500 mL of blood [21], and clinical improvement is expected within 2–3 months [23]. The plasma concentration of ferritin must fall
below $25 \propto g/L$, and hemoglobin must reach a level of 10 g/dL before improvement can be
seen [29]. Although no adverse effects have been reported with its use during pregnancy,
venesection in pregnancy should be avoided if possible [1, 2, 14, 22].

Chloroquine has also been used and can be added in refractory cases [14]. There are
few reports regarding its use in acute exacerbations during pregnancy [14]. In the past,
the use of chloroquine was not advocated, owing to reports of birth defects, including

neurosensory hearing loss, mental retardation, and neonatal convulsions [11, 24], and since it was found to be embryotoxic and teratogenic in rats [14]. However, if the mother's condition is refractory to other measures, chloroquine should be used since the benefits will outweigh the risks [14]. If chloroquine treatment is indicated, ophthalmologic evaluation should be performed before and during treatment to prevent maculopathy [14].

Cesarean section is not indicated in PCT patients. General anesthesia is safe [10] and regional anesthesia can also be used in these patients for labor and operative or normal delivery, as long as a full anesthetic assessment is made [12].

There are too few case reports to accurately judge fetal prognosis in this disease; however, all the patients reported in the literature produced normal infants [28]. However, it is important to assess the newborn in the immediate postpartum period and screen for the presence of PCT, both for genetic purposes and for avoidance of inducing factors in the child [14]. Currently there is not enough information available regarding breast-feeding and PCT [1, 14].

10.2
Acrodermatitis Enteropathica

Acrodermatitis enteropathica was first described by Brandt in 1936 and was named by Danbolt and Closs in 1942 [7, 20]. It is an autosomal recessive disorder characterized by acral and periorificial dermatitis [20].

Acrodermatitis enteropathica is said always to flare during pregnancy, with a measurable decline in serum zinc concentrations beginning early in pregnancy [5, 28]. The decrease in zinc levels is not completely attributed to increased fetal demand for zinc, because levels also decline and the disease flares after oral contraceptive use [28]. Estrogens therefore are thought to play an important primary role [5, 20].

The typical clinical course of acrodermatitis enteropathica patients during pregnancy has been summarized by Bronson et al. [5]. In some patients the diagnosis of the disease is definitively made only when an exacerbation appears during pregnancy, and even then there might be confusion with impetigo herpetiformis or herpes gestationis, unless serum zinc is measured [5]. In the characteristic patient there may be a sporadic, mild, nonspecific skin rash during childhood, which goes into remission at puberty [5]. Diarrhea is slight or absent [5]. During gestation, late in the first or early in the second trimester, the skin disease reappears, with progressive worsening until delivery. Postpartum there is rapid, spontaneous clearing [5].

Most offspring of acrodermatitis enteropathica patients are normal; however, there are single reports of anencephaly [16] and achondroplastic dwarfism, with neonatal death [26], associated with untreated maternal acrodermatitis enteropathica. In addition, zinc deficiency is a known teratogenic substance in mice. Therefore, it is necessary to appropriately diagnose and treat acrodermatitis enteropathica during pregnancy [28]. Zinc supplementation, with the goal of maintaining normal serum zinc levels, seems to be effective in preventing adverse fetal effects and it may also clear the skin manifestations in the mother [4].

10

Summary

› Porphyria cutanea tarda (PCT) may be exacerbated by pregnancy during the first trimester, correlating with a physiologic rise in serum estrogen levels and a high rate of excretion of porphyrins. During the second and third trimesters the skin disease improves.
› Cases of gestational diabetes and preeclampsia have been reported in pregnant PCT patients.
› Management of PCT during pregnancy includes observation and avoidance of alcohol, iron, and exposure to sunlight. Phlebotomies and chloroquine can also be utilized.
› There are no known adverse effects of PCT in the mother on the fetus.
› Acrodermatitis enteropathica always flares during pregnancy, and might be attributable to the direct effect of estrogen.
› Since there are several reports of malformations in the fetus of acrodermatitis enteropathica patients, it is necessary to appropriately diagnose and treat acrodermatitis enteropathica during pregnancy with zinc supplementations.

References

1. Aziz Ibrahim A, Esen UI (2004) Porphyria cutanea tarda in pregnancy: a case report. J Obstet Gynaecol 24:574–575
2. Baxi LV, Rubeo TJ Jr, Katz B et al (1983) Porphyria cutanea tarda and pregnancy. Am J Obstet Gynecol 146:333–334
3. Boyer PJ, Dillon M, Navaie M et al (1994) Factors predictive of maternal-fetal transmission of HIV-1. Preliminary analysis of zidovudine given during pregnancy and/or delivery. JAMA 271:1925–1930
4. Brenton DP, Jackson MJ, Young A (1981) Two pregnancies in a patient with acrodermatitis enteropathica treated with zinc sulphate. Lancet 2:500–502
5. Bronson DM, Barsky R, Barsky S (1983) Acrodermatitis enteropathica. J Am Acad Dermatol 9:140–144
6. Cohen PR, Suarez SM, DeLeo VA (1990) Porphyria cutanea tarda in human immunodeficiency virus-infected patients. JAMA 264:1315–1316
7. Danbolt N (1979) Acrodermatitis enteropathica. Br J Dermatol 100:37–40
8. Gilchrest B, Pathak MA, Parrish JA (1975) Letter: porphyria cutanea tarda in young women. Arch Dermatol 111:263–264
9. Goerz G, Hammer G (1983) Porphyria cutanea tarda and pregnancy. Dermatologica 166:316–318
10. Harrison GG, Meissner PN, Hift RJ (1993) Anaesthesia for the porphyric patient. Anaesthesia 48:417–421
11. Hart CW, Naunton RF (1964) The ototoxicity of chloroquine phosphate. Arch Otolaryngol 80:407–412
12. James MF, Hift RJ (2000) Porphyrias. Br J Anaesth 85:143–153
13. Lamon JM, Frykholm BC (1979) Pregnancy and porphyria cutanea tarda. Johns Hopkins Med J 145:235–237

14. Loret de Mola JR, Muise KL, Duchon MA (1996) Porphyria cutanea tarda and pregnancy. Obstet Gynecol Surv 51:493–497

15. Malina L, Lim CK (1988) Manifestation of familial porphyria cutanea tarda after childbirth. Br J Dermatol 118:243–245

16. Mambidge KM, Neldner KH, Walravens PA (1975) Letter: zinc,acrodermatitis enteropathica, and congenital malformations. Lancet 1:577–578

17. Marks R (1982) Porphyria cutanea tarda. Arch Dermatol 118:452

18. Navas S, Bosch O, Castillo I et al (1995) Porphyria cutanea tarda and hepatitis C and B viruses infection: a retrospective study. Hepatology 21:279–284

19. O'Reilly FM, Darby C, Fogarty J et al (1997) Screening of patients with iron overload to identify hemochromatosis and porphyria cutanea tarda. Arch Dermatol 133:1098–1101

20. Perez-Maldonado A, Kurban AK (2006) Metabolic diseases and pregnancy. Clin Dermatol 24:88–90

21. Perez M, Sanchez JL, Aguilo F (1983) Endocrinologic profile of patients with idiopathic melasma. J Invest Dermatol 81:543–545

22. Rajka G (1984) Pregnancy and porphyria cutanea tarda. Acta Derm Venereol 64:444–445

23. Sarkany RP (2001) The management of porphyria cutanea tarda. Clin Exp Dermatol 26:225–232

24. Tanenbaum L, Tuffanelli DL (1980) Antimalarial agents. Chloroquine, hydroxychloroquine, and quinacrine. Arch Dermatol 116:587–591

25. Urbanek RW, Cohen DJ (1994) Porphyria cutanea tarda: pregnancy versus estrogen effect. J Am Acad Dermatol 31:390–392

26. Vedder JS (1956) Acrodermatitis enteropathica (Danbolt-Closs) in five siblings; efficacy of diodoquin in its management. J Pediatr 48:212–219

27. Waldenstrom J (1937) Studien über Porphyrie. Acta Med Scand 82:1

28. Winton GB (1989) Skin diseases aggravated by pregnancy. J Am Acad Dermatol 20:1–13

29. Yeh SW, Ahmed B, Sami N et al (2003) Blistering disorders: diagnosis and treatment. Dermatol Ther 16:214–223

Pruritus Gravidarum and Intrahepatic Cholestasis of Pregnancy

11

11.1
Definition

Pruritus gravidarum (PG) is a generalized, severe itchiness of late pregnancy where the only skin lesions are those secondary to scratching [74, 88]. It is uncertain whether it is an extension of the physiologic changes ("pregnancy is cholestatic") [79] or a specific dermatosis [1, 88]. It clears at parturition, tends to reappear with consecutive pregnancies, and results from cholestasis in genetically predisposed women [74]. This state is divided by some into those severe cases with jaundice [intrahepatic cholestasis of pregnancy (ICP)] and those with pruritus and biochemical abnormalities, such as elevated levels of serum bile acids, but without hyperbilirubinemia (PG) [78]. The disease results from disturbances of bilirubin excretion by the effects of estrogen and/or progestins [1, 38].

11.2
Introduction

Pruritus is considered by numerous investigators to be one of the most common cutaneous symptoms in pregnancy [86]. According to one author [43], pruritus occurs in at least 18% of pregnant women. Pruritus can stem from many frequent primary causes which are not characteristic to pregnancy such as scabies, trichomonal vaginitis, urticaria, drug eruption, pediculosis, atopic dermatitis, and candida [74]. Other causes of generalized pruritus without primary skin abnormalities are liver disease, renal failure, anemia, diabetes, underlying malignancy, hypothyroidism, and hyperthyroidism [7, 23]. If these causes are eliminated, a small group of patients remains whose pruritus may be related to functional hepatic disturbances and cholestasis [88].

The syndrome of jaundice in late pregnancy was described for the first time by Kehrer [44] in 1907. He associated it with intractable pruritus, which continued until delivery

A. Ingber, *Obstetric Dermatology*,
DOI: 10.1007/978-3-540-88399-9, © Springer-Verlag Berlin Heidelberg 2009

11

and was liable to recur in following pregnancies. Following reports from Arfwedson [6], Svanborg [82], and Thorling [84], this recurrent jaundice of pregnancy was associated with a nonfatal and reversible cholestatic process occurring in certain genetically predisposed women. The development of the percutaneous needle liver biopsy technique and the synthesis of new anabolic and estrogenic steroids, which sometimes reproduced the full syndrome in susceptible individuals, led to the recognition that numerous cases of previously unexplained pruritus of pregnancy were actually an anicteric form of the same disease [74]. The association of jaundice and pregnancy has received many names in the medical literature – intrahepatic cholestasis, idiopathic hepatopathy of pregnancy, idiopathic jaundice of pregnancy, recurrent intrahepatic cholestatic jaundice, recurrent jaundice of pregnancy, and obstetric cholestasis [86].

11.3
Incidence

PG has a worldwide distribution [74]. The incidence varies greatly with reporting criteria and even with seasons [ICP was found to be more frequent in the winter months (November, December, and January)] [68, 78]. The reported incidence varies between 0.02 and 2.4% of pregnancies with wide variation in different countries and ethnic groups [1, 13, 80]. The incidence in Europe ranges from ten to 150 per 10,000 pregnancies [53]. The incidence is much lower in the USA (one in 146 to one in 1,293 deliveries) and Canada (Vancouver, one in 217 deliveries) [13, 68]. There is an especially high incidence in some countries and regions, particularly in Scandinavia (3%), northern Europe, Bolivia, and Chile (Chilean Indians 14%). This geographical distribution was first related to a genetic predisposition to the disease [58, 74], but this increase is now thought to have been caused by dietary factors [69]. The disease is said to be distinctly uncommon in Asians or blacks [78].

Overt jaundice occurs in approximately one in every 1,500 pregnancies [72]. The most common cause of jaundice in pregnancy is not ICP, but rather viral hepatitis. ICP is only as second cause [77], and it is estimated to account for only approximately 20% of cases of obstetric jaundice [78].

There is often a positive family history for that condition in up to 50% of those affected [80], and the incidence is higher in association with twin pregnancies. A Mendelian dominant inheritance associated with the human leukocyte antigen A31 and B8 haplotypes has been proposed [54].

11.4
Clinical Presentation

There is a broad spectrum of clinical presentations [78]. PG begins in the late second to early last trimester of pregnancy in two thirds of cases (mean, 31 weeks) [1, 13, 74], but initial presentation as early as 8 weeks has been reported [78]. The onset coincides with a urinary tract infection in at least 50% of cases [68]. Itchiness tends to be intermittent at first, but later it becomes constant [24, 74]. It may be localized, but usually becomes generalized [60, 86]. Usually the abdomen is the primary site of involvement, with PG later spreading to the entire trunk and distal extremities (particularly palms and soles) (Fig. 11.1) [39, 74, 78, 86]. The intensity ranges from mild to severe [74]. Associated symptoms of fatigue, anorexia, nausea, and vomiting are not uncommon [60,74].

Jaundice can be complicated by subclinical steatorrhea, leading to malabsorption of fat and to weight loss and vitamin K deficiency in severe cases [74]. Symptoms tend to persist for the duration of the pregnancy [78]. They fade away after delivery, but characteristically recur with subsequent pregnancies [58]. Variation in the intensity of pruritus occurs during the course of a single pregnancy or from one pregnancy to another [74].

Despite the intense pruritus especially noted at night, the skin typically shows no primary lesion [74], and the diagnosis of ICP is actually refuted by some authors when cutaneous lesions are present [8]. However, because of the intense pruritus, secondary excoriations are common, particularly on the abdomen [24, 74, 86].

Darker urine and light (clay-colored) stools can be seen in up to 50% of cases, but only 20% of patients develop clinical jaundice, usually within 2–4 weeks of the onset of itching [5]. Unlike pruritus, which may wax and wane, jaundice tends to stabilize shortly

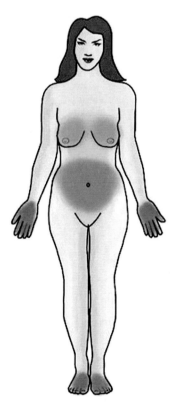

Fig. 11.1 Areas of involvement of pruritus gravidarum

after presentation [78]. The liver may be enlarged and somewhat tender [74]. Some studies have pointed to a higher than normal incidence of cholelithiasis in these patients [30], suggesting that the bile they excrete could be lithogenic because of an abnormal bile acid to cholesterol ratio [3].

11.5
Laboratory Findings

Liver function tests are helpful only in severe cases, as they may give completely normal findings in PG [88]. Increased levels of serum bile acids (particularly cholic acid, but also chenodeoxycholic acid and deoxycholic acid), especially postprandial levels, are regarded as a very sensitive indicator of ICP [50, 52], and demonstrating increased levels of serum bile acids in the absence of alternative explanations essentially confirms the diagnosis [78]. They are typically 3–100 times higher than normal (mean, 1,349 μg/100 mL) [67, 78]. In those without jaundice, elevated levels of serum bile acids may be the only identifiable laboratory abnormality (PG).

Serum levels of direct bilirubin may be normal or slightly elevated, rarely exceeding 2–8 mg/dL [74, 78]. There is elevation of cholesterol, triglycerides, phospholipids, lipoprotein X, alkaline phosphatase, 5 -nucleotidase, leucine aminopeptidase, and γ-glutamyl transpeptidase levels beyond those seen in normal pregnant women [38, 45, 60, 67, 74, 82, 83]. Levels of liver transaminases and lactate dehydrogenase are usually only slightly elevated [5]. It should be noted, however, that alkaline phosphatase, γ-glutamyl transpeptidase, and cholesterol measurements are unreliable during pregnancy. However, aspartate transaminase typically remains within 4 times the normal range, even in those with ICP [78]. Serum abnormalities do not parallel fetal risk and are useful only to confirm the presence or absence of disease [78]. Serum prolactin levels have previously been reported as high in this disease [91]; this has not been confirmed, however [64].

Prothrombin time may be prolonged in very severe cases with complete absence of bile flow and vitamin K malabsorption [74]. Activated partial thromboplastin time may also be prolonged in severe cases [80]. Hepatic ultrasonography findings are normal [78].

11.6
Histopathology

The structure of the skin in PG is usually not specific, and shows epidermal ulceration [14]. In the more severe icteric forms of the disease, percutaneous liver biopsy shows only nonspecific centrilobular cholestasis that can be patchy or mild but that can also be severe, with widely dilated, engorged bile canaliculi with bile thrombi and an overall flooding of parenchyma with bile pigment [68, 74]. The liver parenchyma is otherwise normal with little or no portal inflammatory response [4]. The abnormalities are fully reversible and do not lead to any lasting functional or structural hepatic damage [74]. The changes seen on electron microscopy are similar to those seen in other types of intrahepatic cholestasis, namely, focal dilatation of bile canaliculi containing biliary material and loss or distortion of microvilli [74].

To put it briefly, Haemmerli [33] appropriately stated in 1966 that "cholestasis is clinically marked, biochemically moderate, and histologically minimal."

11.7 Physiopathology

The cause of the cholestasis is unknown [55], and a single biochemical anomaly explaining ICP has yet to be defined [78]. Hormonal, genetic, environmental, and probably alimentary factors play a role in the pathogenesis of the condition [53].

The pruritus is considered to be secondary to an increase in the concentration of bile acids in serum and within the skin [39], and their levels in the serum and in the skin have been correlated by some investigators with the severity of pruritus [14, 49]. It appears that there is a stronger correlation between skin levels than between serum levels [36]. It should be noted, however, that cases with high serum bile acids without pruritus have been reported [68].

The mechanism by which the level of bile acids in the skin produces pruritus is not understood [23]. Varadi [85] studied this mechanism, and produced pruritus by application of pure bile salts in a concentration similar to serum levels in obstructive jaundice. Bile acids may solubilize lipid cellular membranes by their detergent properties, and release histamine and proteolytic enzymes such as lysosomal proteases which affect free nerve endings [36, 85]. However, the concept may be oversimplified since pure synthetic detergents fail to replicate the pruritus [74]. Bile acids might also induce pruritus by a direct effect on the central nervous system or on peripheral nerve endings [36].

The increase in the levels of serum bile acids during pregnancy is connected to a decreased capability for hepatic excretion of organic anions (bilirubin, bile acids, and other compounds) [74]. Certain hormonal changes associated with pregnancy may play an important role in the cause of the condition [86]. Placental estrogens and progestins have been associated with this decrease in hepatic excretory function since the 1950s [74]. Adlercreutz [2] reported that subjects who had suffered from recurrent jaundice in pregnancy developed pruritus and/or jaundice after administration of oral contraceptives. This observation has been confirmed many times subsequently.

The estrogens have been found to be most important, as was suggested by the finding that symptoms and signs are not reproduced when challenge is made with the progesterone part of the oral contraceptive [58]. In addition, estrogens, in particular glucuronides, such as estriol-16α-D-glucuronide and estradiol-17β-glucuronide, have shown cholestatic effects in animal studies [48].

The effect of estrogens was found to be mediated by a direct action on the hepatocyte canalicular membrane [74]. These compounds decrease the sodium-dependent bile acid uptake into hepatocytes and inhibit basolateral transport proteins [15, 81]. A higher incidence of ICP in mothers of patients with progressive familial intrahepatic cholestasis or benign recurrent intrahepatic cholestasis was demonstrated by several studies [16, 87]. Patients with progressive familial intrahepatic cholestasis 3 exhibit mutations of the multidrug resistance 3 gene, which encodes the canalicular phopsphatidylcholine translocase, a transport protein [17]. Furthermore, heterozygosity for the same deletion (1712delT) in the multidrug resistance 3 gene was found in six women with ICP [20, 40]. Thus, the importance of these transport proteins in inducing this disease is reinforced. It has also been hypothesized that estrogens regulate actin molecules, which act intracellularly to mediate bile excretion [66].

Progestins may also have a synergistic effect. The increased levels of pregnanediol and progesterone inhibit the hepatic enzyme glucuronyl transferase, resulting in impaired conjugation and excretion of bilirubin which causes intrahepatic cholestasis [35], and also in delayed clearance of estrogen and amplification of its effects [3]. Additionally, the increased levels of sulfated progesterone metabolites in the serum may saturate the maximal transport capacity of membrane transport proteins of the hepatocyte [53, 59]. Synthetic progestogens of the 19-norprogestogen group are converted to estrogen in measurable quantities, thus leading to a direct effect on hepatocyte cells [74]. Finally, progesterone might also have a direct effect by itself, as it has been shown to bind to and regulate the activity of multidrug-resistance translocases [18].

One hypothesis is that the relative fall in hepatic blood flow during pregnancy leads to a decreased clearance of estrogens that results in an increase in biliary cholesterol concentration and secretion, and also impairs the capacity of the liver to transport anions, such as bilirubin and bile salts [72]. Whether the abovementioned abnormalities are causal or secondary to cholestasis is unknown [47].

11.8
Diagnosis

The diagnosis is clinical, but laboratory tests are important to support it and exclude other conditions [68]. The previously mentioned coincidental causes of pruritus in pregnancy can be differentiated from PG by history, physical examination, and appropriate microscopic examinations for candidiasis, scabies, pediculosis, or vaginal trichomoniasis [88].

If jaundice is present, other causes of hyperbilirubinemia have to be excluded [74]. Viral or toxic hepatitis can usually be ruled out by the absence of marked transaminase elevation (greater than 5 times elevation) and appropriate serologic tests, and marked systemic symptoms [74, 78, 88]. Choledocholithiasis is unlikely in the absence of elevated levels of urinary urobilinogen, biliary abdominal pain, fever, leukocytosis, and hepatomegaly [74, 88]. Hemolysis is a rare cause of jaundice in pregnancy [74].

The clinical picture is strikingly similar to that of drug-induced jaundice (e.g., chlorpromazine, thorazine, grisefulvin, sulfanilamide, indomethacin, and methyltestosterone), with a histologic picture of intrahepatic cholestasis and little evidence of other hepatocellular damage [58, 88]. However, removal of all potentially offending drugs will lead to prompt resolution [88].

There is, by definition, no primary dermatitis associated with ICP, but only the secondary findings of excoriations and scratch papules [78]. The finding of cutaneous inflammation should incite a search for other causes [78]. Failure of pruritus to stop within days of delivery or the persistence of elevated live functions tests should prompt one to exclude primary biliary cirrhosis [78]. This disease can be evaluated using tests for autoantibodies [77].

In rare situations when further information is needed for a specific diagnosis, liver biopsy is probably safe in pregnancy as in the nonpregnant state [11, 88]. Ultrasonography has been of some help in the detection of stones and dilated bile ducts in extrahepatic obstruction [74]. Some methods of investigation, such as transhepatic cholangiography or endoscopic retrograde cholangiography, are unacceptable because of radiation risk to the fetus [11].

11.9
Treatment

Treatment of ICP is symptomatic and directed at controlling the pruritus [60, 78]. Mild attacks need only reassurance and simple bland, antipruritic preparations such as soothing oatmeal baths or cooling lotions such as menthol in aqueous cream. Emollients, primrose oil, calamine lotion, and weak topical corticosteroid ointment can also be used [22, 25, 42, 74, 78, 88, 90]. Epomediol and silymarine may be helpful in controlling the pruritus in mild ICP [32, 47]. S-Denosyl-D-methionine has been shown to have beneficial effects on both pruritus and biochemical alterations in patients with mild ICP [28]. Activated charcoal had also limited success [57]. It is helpful to avoid anxiety, fatigue, and irritating clothing [90]. Rest and a low-fat diet have ameliorated symptoms in some patients [68]. The patient should be reassured that this condition is temporary, and that rapid resolution will usually occur at parturition [86].

If ICP is severe, therapy with ion-exchange resins, such as cholestyramine, should be introduced [35]. Cholestyramine is a nonabsorbable, synthetic ion-exchange resin which strongly binds bile acids in the gut, removing them from enterohepatic circulation when complete obstruction of the biliary tree is not present [74]. Dosages of 4 g two to three times a day have produced a reduction in serum bile acid levels and a relief from pruritus in some patients [49]. Varying degrees of success have been reported with this regimen [14]. Small uncontrolled trials indicate that cholestyramine may be effective in half of patients with mild ICP [34, 49]. Another trial showed a clinical response in 70% of patients [63]. Nonetheless, its use is still in dispute because of the lack of placebo-controlled cholestyramine trials, which makes it difficult to asses its effectiveness [48]. Cholestyramine has several drawbacks which include that it may be futile in severe ICP, it needs to be administered for several days before pruritus is improved, and it does not affect the biochemical abnormalities of ICP [46, 49, 57, 68, 76]. Cholestyramine may precipitate vitamin K, and thus lead to coagulopathy [46, 53]. A severe case of fetal intracranial hemorrhage during cholestyramine therapy has been reported [73]. Side effects are frequent but minor – many patients find the medication distasteful and complain that it causes nausea, bloating, abdominal cramps, and constipation [74].

The use of ursodeoxycholic acid (UDCA) has recently gained favor [78]. This hydrophilic bile acid, normally present in small concentrations, is thought to replace other, more hydrophobic and cytotoxic bile salts in the cycle of enterohepatic circulation and sulfated progesterone metabolites [53, 78]. UDCA was found to reduce bile acid levels in cord blood, amniotic fluid, and colostrum [10, 56]. The recommended dosage is 15 mg/kg per day [68], and its daily use for 3 weeks controls both the pruritus and the biochemical abnormalities [62]. This was confirmed by the results of four randomized UDCA trails [19, 27, 61, 62]. UDCA works faster than cholestyramine and has a more persistent effect on pruritus [48]. Its effect may be increased by its coadministration with S-adenosylme-thionine [61]. UDCA is safe for mother and fetus [19, 27, 61, 62]. Its use has been reported not only to control symptoms, but also to decrease any risk of adverse fetal outcome, including premature labor, fetal distress, and fetal death [65, 69].

There are authors who have successfully treated ICP with oral corticosteroids [37]. Twelve milligrams of dexamethasone daily for 6 days has been used with suppression of fetoplacental estrogen production and resolution of pruritic symptoms in a small uncontrolled trial [37]. There is also a report of ACTH use in cases of intractable pruritus [86].

Nonerythemogenic UVB radiation 3–5 days a week is sometimes successful in treating intractable pruritus [89, 92]. Another therapeutic preparation that has been evaluated is oral guar gum. It is a gel-forming dietary fiber that increases the elimination of bile acids, stabilizes serum levels, and decreases pruritic complaints by patients [70].

Phenobarbital has been found to promote enhanced bile excretion in cholestatic liver disease [9]. Its mechanism of action is related to its ability to enhance the catabolism of the bile salts by inducing the hepatic cytochrome system [77]. High dosages (10 mg/kg per day) have to be used, however, and somnolence seriously limits its usefulness [9]. In addi-tion, the high doses required may be contraindicated in pregnancy because of unknown effects on the fetus [11].

Antihistamines are a modality that is reasonably safe [88]. Studies of their teratogenic potential show that diphenhydramine, azatadine, cyclizine, tripelennamine, cyprohepta-dine, dexchlorpheniramine, dymenhydrinate, doxylamine, meclicine, pheniramine, and chlorpheniramine are apparently safe during pregnancy [60, 88]. Brompheniramine is sus-pect for significant teratogenic potential [88], and thus it is best avoided during pregnancy [88]. Antihistamines offer little help, and thus may probably be used only as adjunctive therapy [74, 88].

Vitamin K supplements should be given whenever jaundice is of long duration, the prothrombin time is prolonged, or when cholestyramine is employed because the drug also binds fat-soluble vitamins [14, 74]. The prothrombin time should be routinely monitored, and intramuscular vitamin K administered as necessary [78].

11.10
Prognosis

Delivery rapidly brings rapid disappearance of the symptoms and restoration of normal liver function and structure [74, 88]. To date, there have been no reports of permanent liver damage [86]. Pruritus usually subsides within 24–48 h of delivery, but may continue for up to 2 weeks [13, 74, 78]. Jaundice usually disappears within the same period, but may last for up to 4 weeks [74]. The bile salt levels return to normal in 4–6 weeks [77].

PG may recur 40–70% of the time with variable severity in subsequent pregnancies [47, 78, 88]. Recurrences also occur with the use of estrogen-containing medications [88]. No detectable abnormalities are generally present between gestations [78]. Intervening symptom-free pregnancies have been reported [1].

The prognosis for the mother is excellent [86]. Maternal morbidity is limited to the inconvenience caused by the pruritus and the potential for malabsorption [74, 78], but serious bleeding aberrations such as postpartum uterine hemorrhage may occur in patients who have abnormal clotting times owing to reduction of vitamin K [78]. In a 15-year follow-up study there was found to be an increased incidence of subsequent cholelithiasis or gallbladder disease in this group of patients [29, 78].

The reports concerning fetal morbidity and mortality are conflicting [86]. Some investigators believe that the fetus is unaffected [4, 39, 76]. In 1982, Shaw et al. [76] reported no increased fetal deaths; however, these results are in dispute, since the investigators instituted frequent surveillance (daily nonstress tests) early in the third trimester, and they delivered the babies once fetal lung maturity had been documented by amniocentesis [76].

Others believe that there is an increase in fetal mortality [21]. In the series of 56 pregnancies of Reid et al. [65], six intrauterine or neonatal deaths were reported. The most common cause of the increased perinatal mortality was prematurity and stillbirth [65]. The patients with the more severe and cholestatic disease had the most increased risk of prematurity and stillbirth [65]. A prospective cohort study established a correlation between bile acid levels and fetal complications, with a statistically significant increase in adverse fetal outcomes reported in patients with bile acid levels of 16.34 µg/mL (40 µmol/L) or more [31]; however, perinatal death did occur in women with only pruritus [65]. Fisk and Storey [26] reported on 83 pregnancies complicated by cholestasis. The incidence of meconium-stained amniotic fluid was 45%, intrapartum distress occurred in 22% of cases, and there were two stillbirths in this series [26].

There is uniformity in reports that the incidence of prematurity, low-birth-weight babies, intrauterine asphyxia, and postpartum hemorrhage is significantly increased in pregnancies complicated by frank obstetric cholestasis [21, 29, 39, 41]. These probably stem from placental anoxia [51]. Assessment of the placenta often reveals nonspecific abnormalities (degenerative changes, edematous villi, infarcts), which may contribute to fetal hypoxia [51]. Decreased fetal elimination of toxic bile acids may cause vasoconstriction of placental chorionic veins in vitro and meconium passage [75, 76]. Meconium can cause acute umbilical vein constriction [12].

Most authors recommend management of these patients in a center fully equipped for high-risk pregnancies, and early cardiotocographic fetal monitoring and the induction of labor in week 38 of gestation in mild cases and in week 36 of gestation in severe cases [71]. Some authors, however, advocate the assessment of lung maturity and delivery if a patient is at 36 weeks or more of gestation and if the cervix is favorable, but recommend pharmacologic treatment if the patient is at less than 36 weeks of gestation [32]. Others suggest that the frequency of fetal surveillance should correlate with the intensity of laboratory abnormalities and patient symptoms [77]. The cost-effectiveness of these protocols has not been determined [48].

11

Summary

> Pruritus gravidarum is a state of wide clinical variety, which may be an extension of a physiologic pruritic state. In its severe form it presents as jaundice.
> Incidence is variable, with higher incidence in Chile and northern Europe.
> Clinical presentation of severe pruritus is in the third trimester, with no primary skin lesions. Secondary excoriations are common.
> Laboratory findings show abnormal liver function and elevated levels of serum bile acids.
> This state originates from the effects of estrogen and progesterone on the bile acid excretion properties of the hepatocytes.
> In mild cases treatment is with emollients. More severe cases respond to ion-exchange resins and UV therapy.
> Maternal prognosis is excellent. There is an increased rate for fetal distress, stillbirth, and preterm delivery. Strict surveillance and early induction is recommended.

References

1. (1975) Editorial: itching in pregnancy. Br Med J 3:608
2. Adlercreutz H (1964) Oral contraceptives and liver damage. Br Med J 2:1133
3. Adlercreutz H, Tenhunen R (1970) Some aspects of the interaction between natural and synthetic female sex hormones and the liver. Am J Med 49:630–648
4. Adlercreutz H, Svanborg A, Anberg A (1967) Recurrent jaundice in pregnancy. II. A study of the estrogens and their conjugation in late pregnancy. Am J Med 42:341–347
5. Al-Fares SI, Jones SV, Black MM (2001) The specific dermatoses of pregnancy: a re-appraisal. J Eur Acad Dermatol Venereol 15:197–206
6. Arfwedson H (1956) General pruritus in pregnancy; symptom of liver dysfunction. Obstet Gynecol 7:274–276
7. Barankin B, Silver SG, Carruthers A (2002) The skin in pregnancy. J Cutan Med Surg 6:236–240
8. Berg B, Helm G, Petersohn L et al (1986) Cholestasis of pregnancy. Clinical and laboratory studies. Acta Obstet Gynecol Scand 65:107–113
9. Bloomer JR, Boyer JL (1975) Phenobarbital effects in cholestatic liver diseases. Ann Intern Med 82:310–317
10. Brites D, Rodrigues CM (1998) Elevated levels of bile acids in colostrum of patients with cholestasis of pregnancy are decreased following ursodeoxycholic acid therapy [see comments]. J Hepatol 29:743–751
11. Bynum TE (1977) Hepatic and gastrointestinal disorders in pregnancy. Med Clin North Am 61:129–138
12. Campos GA, Guerra FA, Israel EJ (1986) Effects of cholic acid infusion in fetal lambs. Acta Obstet Gynecol Scand 65:23–26
13. Cohen LM (1998) Dermatoses of pregnancy. West J Med 169:223–224
14. Dacus JV (1990) Pruritus in pregnancy. Clin Obstet Gynecol 33:738–745
15. Davis RA, Kern F Jr, Showalter R et al (1978) Alterations of hepatic Na+, K+-ATPase and bile flow by estrogen: effects on liver surface membrane lipid structure and function. Proc Natl Acad Sci USA 75:4130–4134

16. de Pagter AG, van Berge Henegouwen GP, ten Bokkel Huinink JA et al (1976) Familial benign recurrent intrahepatic cholestasis. Interrelation with intrahepatic cholestasis of pregnancy and from oral contraceptives? Gastroenterology 71:202–207

17. de Vree JM, Jacquemin E, Sturm E et al (1998) Mutations in the MDR3 gene cause progressive familial intrahepatic cholestasis. Proc Natl Acad Sci USA 95:282–287

18. Debry P, Nash EA, Neklason DW et al (1997) Role of multidrug resistance P-glycoproteins in cholesterol esterification. J Biol Chem 272:1026–1031

19. Diaferia A, Nicastri PL, Tartagni M et al (1996) Ursodeoxycholic acid therapy in pregnant women with cholestasis. Int J Gynaecol Obstet 52:133–140

20. Dixon PH, Weerasekera N, Linton KJ et al (2000) Heterozygous MDR3 missense mutation associated with intrahepatic cholestasis of pregnancy: evidence for a defect in protein trafficking. Hum Mol Genet 9:1209–1217

21. Eliakim M, Sadovsky E, Stein O et al (1966) Recurrent cholestatic jaundice of pregnancy. Report of five cases and electron microscopic observations. Arch Intern Med 117:696–705

22. Elling SV, Powell FC (1997) Physiological changes in the skin during pregnancy. Clin Dermatol 15:35–43

23. Errickson CV, Matus NR (1994) Skin disorders of pregnancy. Am Fam Physician 49:605–610

24. Eudy SF, Baker GF (1990) Dermatopathology for the obstetrician. Clin Obstet Gynecol 33:728–737

25. Fagan EA (1994) Intrahepatic cholestasis of pregnancy. BMJ 309:1243–1244

26. Fisk NM, Storey GN (1988) Fetal outcome in obstetric cholestasis. Br J Obstet Gynaecol 95:1137–1143

27. Floreani A, Paternoster D, Melis A et al (1996) S-Adenosylmethionine versus ursodeoxycholic acid in the treatment of intrahepatic cholestasis of pregnancy: preliminary results of a controlled trial. Eur J Obstet Gynecol Reprod Biol 67:109–113

28. Frezza M, Surrenti C, Manzillo G et al (1990) Oral S-adenosylmethionine in the symptomatic treatment of intrahepatic cholestasis. A double-blind, placebo-controlled study. Gastroenterology 99:211–215

29. Furhoff AK (1974) Itching in pregnancy. A 15-year follow-up study. Acta Med Scand 196:403–410

30. Furhoff AK, Hellstrom K (1974) Jaundice in pregnancy. A follow-up study of the series of women originally reported by L. Thorling. II. Present health of the women. Acta Med Scand 196:181–189

31. Glantz A, Marschall HU, Mattsson LA (2004) Intrahepatic cholestasis of pregnancy: Relationships between bile acid levels and fetal complication rates. Hepatology 40:467–474

32. Gonzalez M, Iglesias J, Tiribelli C et al (1992) Symptomatic effect of epomediol in patients with cholestasis of pregnancy. Rev Med Chil 120:545–551

33. Haemmerli U (1966) Jaundice during pregnancy, with special emphasis on recurrent jaundice during pregnancy and its differential diagnosis,. Acta Med Scand 179(Suppl):4

34. Heikkinen J, Maentausta O, Ylostalo P et al (1982) Serum bile acid levels in intrahepatic cholestasis of pregnancy during treatment with phenobarbital or cholestyramine. Eur J Obstet Gynecol Reprod Biol 14:153–162

35. Hellreich P (1974) The skin changes of pregnancy. Cutis 13:82–86

36. Herndon JH Jr (1972) Pathophysiology of pruritus associated with elevated bile acid levels in serum. Arch Intern Med 130:632–637

37. Hirvioja ML, Tuimala R, Vuori J (1992) The treatment of intrahepatic cholestasis of pregnancy by dexamethasone. Br J Obstet Gynaecol 99:109–111

38. Holzbach RT (1976) Jaundice in pregnancy – 1976. Am J Med 61:367–376

39. Holzbach RT, Sanders JH (1965) Recurrent intrahepatic cholestasis of pregnancy: observations on pathogenesis. JAMA 193:542–544

40. Jacquemin E, Cresteil D, Manouvrier S et al (1999) Heterozygous non-sense mutation of the MDR3 gene in familial intrahepatic cholestasis of pregnancy. Lancet 353:210–211
41. Johnston WG, Baskett TF (1979) Obstetric cholestasis. A 14 year review. Am J Obstet Gynecol 133:299–301
42. Jones SV, Black M (1999) Pregnancy dermatoses. J Am Acad Dermatol 40:233–241
43. Kasdon SC (1953) Abdominal pruritus in pregnancy. Am J Obstet Gynecol 65:320–324
44. Kehrer E (1907) Die Bedeutung des Ikterus in der Schwangerscaht für Mutter und Kind. Klinische und experimentelle Untersuchungen. Arch Gynaek 81:129
45. Kreek MJ, Sleisenger MH, Jeffries GH (1967) Recurrent cholestatic jaundice of pregnancy with demonstrated estrogen sensitivity. Am J Med 43:795–803
46. Kroumpouzos G (2002) Intrahepatic cholestasis of pregnancy: what's new. J Eur Acad Dermatol Venereol 16:316–318
47. Kroumpouzos G, Cohen LM (2001) Dermatoses of pregnancy. J Am Acad Dermatol 45:1–19; quiz 19–22
48. Kroumpouzos G, Cohen LM (2003) Specific dermatoses of pregnancy: an evidence-based systematic review. Am J Obstet Gynecol 188:1083–1092
49. Laatikainen T (1978) Effect of cholestyramine and phenobarbital on pruritus and serum bile acid levels in cholestasis of pregnancy. Am J Obstet Gynecol 132:501–506
50. Laatikainen T (1978) Postprandial serum bile acids in cholestasis of pregnancy. Ann Clin Res 10:307–312
51. Laatikainen T, Ikonen E (1977) Serum bile acids in cholestasis of pregnancy. Obstet Gynecol 50:313–318
52. Laatikainen T, Tulenheimo A (1984) Maternal serum bile acid levels and fetal distress in cholestasis of pregnancy. Int J Gynaecol Obstet 22:91–94
53. Lammert F, Marschall HU, Glantz A et al (2000) Intrahepatic cholestasis of pregnancy: molecular pathogenesis, diagnosis and management. J Hepatol 33:1012–1021
54. Lunzer MR (1989) Jaundice in pregnancy. Baillieres Clin Gastroenterol 3:467–483
55. Martin AG, Leal-Khouri S (1992) Physiologic skin changes associated with pregnancy. Int J Dermatol 31:375–378
56. Mazzella G, Rizzo N, Azzaroli F et al (2001) Ursodeoxycholic acid administration in patients with cholestasis of pregnancy: effects on primary bile acids in babies and mothers. Hepatology 33:504–508
57. McDonald JA (1999) Cholestasis of pregnancy. J Gastroenterol Hepatol 14:515–518
58. McKenzie AW (1971) Skin disorders in pregnancy. Practitioner 206:773–780
59. Meng LJ, Reyes H, Axelson M et al (1997) Progesterone metabolites and bile acids in serum of patients with intrahepatic cholestasis of pregnancy: effect of ursodeoxycholic acid therapy. Hepatology 26:1573–1579
60. Murray JC (1990) Pregnancy and the skin. Dermatol Clin 8:327–334
61. Nicastri PL, Diaferia A, Tartagni M et al (1998) A randomised placebo-controlled trial of ursodeoxycholic acid and S-adenosylmethionine in the treatment of intrahepatic cholestasis of pregnancy. Br J Obstet Gynaecol 105:1205–1207
62. Palma J, Reyes H, Ribalta J et al (1997) Ursodeoxycholic acid in the treatment of cholestasis of pregnancy: a randomized, double-blind study controlled with placebo. J Hepatol 27:1022–1028
63. Rampone A, Rampone B, Tirabasso S et al (2002) Prurigo gestationis. J Eur Acad Dermatol Venereol 16:425–426
64. Ranta T, Unnerus HA, Rossi J et al (1979) Elevated plasma prolactin concentration in cholestasis of pregnancy. Am J Obstet Gynecol 134:1–3
65. Reid R, Ivey KJ, Rencoret RH et al (1976) Fetal complications of obstetric cholestasis. Br Med J 1:870–872

11

66. Reyes-Romero MA (1990) Are changes in expression of actin genes involved in estrogen-induced cholestasis? Med Hypotheses 32:39–43
67. Reyes H (1982) The enigma of intrahepatic cholestasis of pregnancy: lessons from Chile. Hepatology 2:87–96
68. Reyes H (1992) The spectrum of liver and gastrointestinal disease seen in cholestasis of pregnancy. Gastroenterol Clin North Am 21:905–921
69. Reyes H (1997) Review: intrahepatic cholestasis. A puzzling disorder of pregnancy. J Gastroenterol Hepatol 12:211–216
70. Riikonen S, Savonius H, Gylling H et al (2000) Oral guar gum, a gel-forming dietary fiber relieves pruritus in intrahepatic cholestasis of pregnancy. Acta Obstet Gynecol Scand 79:260–264
71. Rioseco AJ, Ivankovic MB, Manzur A et al (1994) Intrahepatic cholestasis of pregnancy: a retrospective case-control study of perinatal outcome. Am J Obstet Gynecol 170:890–895
72. Rustgi VK (1989) Liver disease in pregnancy. Med Clin North Am 73:1041–1046
73. Sadler LC, Lane M, North R (1995) Severe fetal intracranial haemorrhage during treatment with cholestyramine for intrahepatic cholestasis of pregnancy. Br J Obstet Gynaecol 102:169–170
74. Sasseville D, Wilkinson RD, Schnader JY (1981) Dermatoses of pregnancy. Int J Dermatol 20:223–241
75. Sepulveda WH, Gonzalez C, Cruz MA et al (1991) Vasoconstrictive effect of bile acids on isolated human placental chorionic veins. Eur J Obstet Gynecol Reprod Biol 42:211–215
76. Shaw D, Frohlich J, Wittmann BA et al (1982) A prospective study of 18 patients with cholestasis of pregnancy. Am J Obstet Gynecol 142:621–625
77. Sherard GB 3rd, Atkinson SM Jr (2001) Focus on primary care: pruritic dermatological conditions in pregnancy. Obstet Gynecol Surv 56:427–432
78. Shornick JK (1998) Dermatoses of pregnancy. Semin Cutan Med Surg 17:172–181
79. Simcock MJ, Forster FM (1967) Pregnancy is cholestatic. Med J Aust 2:971–973
80. Sodhi VK, Sausker WF (1988) Dermatoses of pregnancy. Am Fam Physician 37:131–138
81. Stieger B, Fattinger K, Madon J et al (2000) Drug- and estrogen-induced cholestasis through inhibition of the hepatocellular bile salt export pump (Bsep) of rat liver. Gastroenterology 118:422–430
82. Svanborg A (1954) A study of recurrent jaundice in pregnancy. Acta Obstet Gynecol Scand 33:434–444
83. Svanborg A, Ohlsson S (1959) Recurrent jaundice of pregnancy; a clinical study of twenty-two cases. Am J Med 27:40–49
84. Thorling L (1955) Jaundice in pregnancy; a clinical study. Acta Med Scand Suppl 302:1–123
85. Varadi DP (1974) Pruritus induced by crude bile and purified bile acids. Experimental production of pruritus in human skin. Arch Dermatol 109:678–681
86. Wade TR, Wade SL, Jones HE (1978) Skin changes and diseases associated with pregnancy. Obstet Gynecol 52:233–242
87. Whitington PF, Freese DK, Alonso EM et al (1994) Clinical and biochemical findings in progressive familial intrahepatic cholestasis. J Pediatr Gastroenterol Nutr 18:134–141
88. Winton GB, Lewis CW (1982) Dermatoses of pregnancy. J Am Acad Dermatol 6:977–998
89. Wong RC, Ellis CN (1984) Physiologic skin changes in pregnancy. J Am Acad Dermatol 10:929–940
90. Wong RC, Ellis CN (1989) Physiologic skin changes in pregnancy. Semin Dermatol 8:7–11
91. Ylikorkala O (1973) Maternal serum HPL levels in normal and complicated pregnancy as an index of placental function. Acta Obstet Gynecol Scand Suppl 26:1–52
92. Zoberman E, Farmer ER (1981) Pruritic folliculitis of pregnancy. Arch Dermatol 117:20–22

Herpes (Pemphigoid) Gestationis

12

12.1
Definition

Herpes gestationis (HG), a rare, hormonally mediated, autoimmune disease, is the most clearly defined of the dermatoses of pregnancy [99]. It is characterized by intensely pruritic, recurrent, vesiculobullous eruption in all trimesters of pregnancy characterized by destruction of the epidermal basement membrane through deposition of C3 and a special antibody, the "HG factor" [2, 48, 91, 112]. This condition is the most dramatic and serious of pregnancy eruptions [74]. Genes that provide enhanced susceptibility have been identified, but their specific role in pathogenesis has not been defined [95].

12.2
Introduction

This eruption was first described by Bunel [8] in 1811, and later in the nineteenth century was also reported by Milton [75] and Duhring [21]. Milton in 1872 carefully described the entity and condensed its name from "herpes circinatus bullosus seu gestationis" to the name that was subsequently common: herpes gestationis (HG) [35, 75].

The term "herpes gestationis" is somewhat of a misnomer in that herpes gestationis is not a viral disease [24]. Although a few patients may demonstrate characteristic groupings of herpetiform vesicular lesions at some stage in their disease, there is no evidence of a viral cause [19, 113]. The term "herpes" comes from the Greek word meaning "to creep" and was first applied to skin disease by Galenus in 200 AD. It was used in the past to describe any of the vesicular skin diseases [24] and this is the reason that the vesicular skin disease specifically associated with pregnancy was dubbed "herpes gestationis" [24].

A. Ingber, *Obstetric Dermatology*,
DOI: 10.1007/978-3-540-88399-9, © Springer-Verlag Berlin Heidelberg 2009

HG was considered in the past to be a variant of pemphigus, dermatitis herpeti-formis, and erythema multiforme [91]. At one time, the eruption was even thought to be an allergic reaction to the products of conception [19]. However, extensive laboratory work, which included electron microscopy studies by Pierard et al. [83] and Schaumburg-Lever et al. [94], as well as the application of sensitive immunofluorescence techniques by Provost and Tomasi [85], Jablonska et al. [49], Bushkell et al. [10], and Kocsis et al. [64] have discovered the ultrastructure and mode of production of this disease, and have shown that this entity bears a close resemblance to bullous pemphigoid (BP) [71, 74, 91]; therefore, in 1982, Holmes and Black [41] proposed that the disorder should be named "pemphigus gestationis." Although this is now the preferred term in the UK and Europe, it is used very little in the USA, where it is usually named "herpes gestationis" [2].

12.3
Incidence

By definition, HG is restricted to women of childbearing age, and has been described in women between the ages of 16 and 39 [33, 58, 113]. The exact incidence is unknown [11], and a vast variance in the incidence of the disease has been reported.

The first reports described incidences of approximately one in 3,000–5,000 pregnancies [36, 89]; however, later reports have described a much lower incidence – the incidence of HG in North America was estimated as one in 50,000 pregnancies [114] and in the UK as one in 40,000 pregnancies [4]. Kolodny [65] found that it occurred in only one in 60,000 pregnancies. Others have thought that it is even less common, with an incidence of one per 112,769 deliveries [97]. On the other hand, there are new reports describing a much higher incidence – Roger et al. [88] reported an incidence of one in 1,600 pregnancies and Zurn et al. [116] found an incidence of one in 7,000 pregnancies, suggesting that the incidence of HG may be underestimated. The higher incidences have been related to referral bias, clinical overlap between mild HG and polymorphous eruption of pregnancy, and the inclusion of cases that do not meet the immunologic diagnostic criteria [93, 114, 116]. Whether immunofluorescence testing of all pregnant women with a pruritic dermatosis is reasonable and cost-effective or not remains controversial [30, 31, 93]. In spite of this debatable incidence rate, it is still probably the least common of the specific dermatoses of pregnancy [41].

HG is most common among white subjects, although sporadic occurrences in black women have been reported [105]. There is a higher frequency of human leukocyte antigen (HLA)-DR3, HLA-DR4, or both in patients with the disease [45, 102]. White patients have an increased frequency of either or both HLA-DR3 and HLA-DR4 [26], and the low frequency of HLA-DR4 among African-Americans may explain the relative rarity of HG in this population [26].

In some instances, it has occurred in multiparous patients after a change in consorts [39]; however, an association between a change in partner and the development of HG has not been found in other studies [52, 104].

12.4
Clinical Presentation

The phase of pregnancy at which HG begins varies significantly from patient to patient [45]. It commonly begins between the 12th and 24th weeks of pregnancy (mean onset, 21 weeks) [66, 68, 74], but may occur at any time during pregnancy [36], and also in the puerperium for the first time in 25% of cases [36, 65, 68, 74, 104]. Lawley et al. [68] reported a series of 41 immunologically proven cases of HG, and the onset varied, with eight cases beginning in the first trimester, 15 cases in the second trimester, 12 cases in the third trimester, and six cases immediately postpartum.

It may begin in the first, second, or any pregnancy [36]; however, in a national survey including 24 patients conducted by Holmes et al. [45], most patients were multigravida when they had their first episode of HG. Once established, the course is usually one of exacerbations and remissions, each occurring at intervals of several days to weeks [36, 91]. In 75% of patients there is spontaneous resolution between the 33rd and 40th weeks of gestation [36, 74, 99]. This relative remission in the last weeks of pregnancy may be followed in 75–80% of cases by a rapid flare immediately after delivery [45, 97]. According to Shornick [97] "postpartum onset is often explosive and may occur within hours of delivery."

Those cases which start near the beginning of pregnancy usually cease at or soon after delivery, while the late-onset cases may carry on for a few weeks postpartum [91]. The bullous eruption may clear in 4 weeks postpartum, and the urticarial lesions in 60 weeks [45]. The postpartum duration of HG may increase with the number of involved pregnancies [44] – the postpartum duration of the disease, on average, was 12 weeks after the first involved pregnancy and 31 weeks after the second [46]. Breast-feeding has a propensity to shorten this duration [46]. With breast-feeding, the average time for lesions to resolve was found by Holmes et al. [46] to be 5 weeks for bullous lesions and 24 weeks for urticarial lesions, in comparison with 24 and 68 weeks, respectively, for women who do not breast-feed. However, the effects of breast-feeding and prolactin on HG merit further investigation [67].

There are reports of cases in which the disease activity has persisted for several years postpartum [41], and in two cases conversion to BP was reported [51]. It has been suggested that systemic steroid therapy may be the cause of this tendency toward increased duration of the disease [13]. According to the author's experience, in most of the HG pregnancies the fetus is male.

In some instances repeated minor relapses arise over the next 9–18 months in association with menstruation and ovulation [35, 36, 74, 91]. When the disorder has occurred in pregnancy, the prescription of oral contraceptives is likely to precipitate a similar eruption in 20–50% of cases [56, 76]. This is true when use of oral contraceptives had been started between 1 and 5 months after delivery of an involved gestation [97]. Therefore, hormonal contraception is contraindicated in patients with HG [2]. This association with oral contraceptives supports the theory that estrogens alone may promote recurrence but not set off the disease [96]. Onset of the disease was also seen with hydatidiform mole [22] or choriocarcinoma [110].

Recurrence in subsequent pregnancies is the rule [76]. Although it has often been said that it tends to be more severe and begin earlier in succeeding pregnancies, there is no evidence that it is so [36, 46, 99, 104]. Less commonly, it may skip pregnancies [56], and there have been well-documented reports of skipped pregnancies in 8% of patients with HG [46, 48, 52, 98, 104]. This cannot be predicted by any clinical, epidemiologic, or laboratory features [46, 104]. Shornick [97] found that most women who are faced with the high reappearance rate of HG ask for sterilization. As a result, it is necessary that the correct diagnosis is made when the disease first occurs [97].

The clinical profile is vastly variable [95]. In some patients there is limited involvement, while others have extensive lesions [95]. In addition, in a given patient, the clinical manifestations may vary in intensity from one pregnancy to another [95]. Prodromal symptoms (malaise, nausea, headache, hot and cold sensations, constipation, fever and chills) often herald the onset of the eruption for several days or weeks in severe cases [36, 112, 113]. Preceding symptoms of severe generalized itching and burning sensations are prominent features of the disease [24, 35, 36, 91]. These are followed by the development of papulovesicles and subepidermal bullae [74]. The eruption is quite polymorphous and usually begins with areas of patchy erythema and subcutaneous edema. The edematous plaques are usually symmetrically distributed, and have a predilection for the trunk, especially the abdomen, thighs, palms, and soles (Figs. 12.1–12.8) [19, 45, 113]. In half of all cases, lesions begin on the abdomen, often within or immediately next to the umbilicus

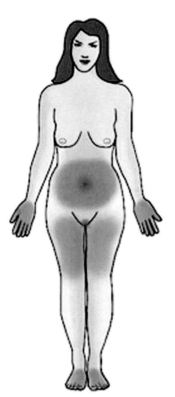

Fig. 12.1 Areas of involvement of herpes gestationis, anterior view

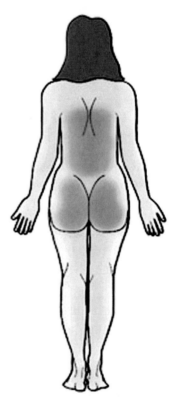

Fig. 12.2 Areas of involvement of herpes gestationis, posterior view

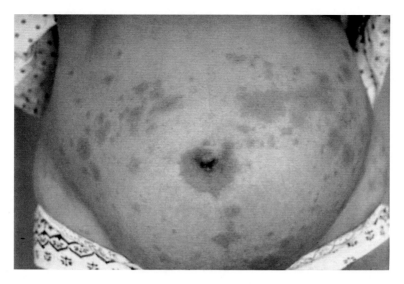

Fig. 12.3 Herpes gestationis. Typical lesions: vesicles on edematous erythemic skin, arranged in a herpetiform pattern. Note typical umbilical involvement

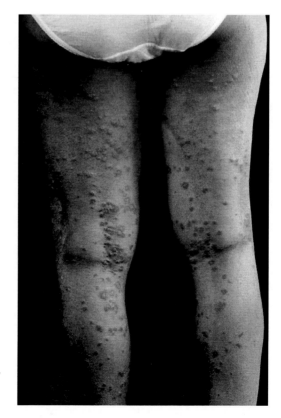

Fig. 12.4 Herpes gestationis. Numerous grouped vesicles on the lower limbs

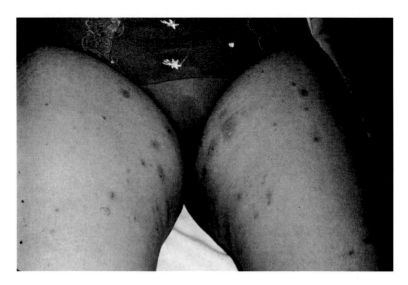

Fig. 12.5 Herpes gestationis. Close view of typical edematous lesions and vesicles on the thighs

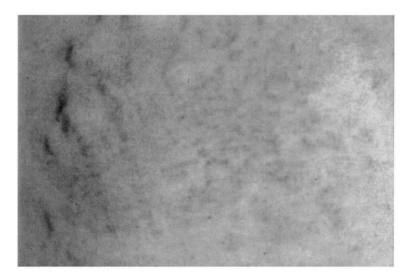

Fig. 12.6 Herpes gestationis. Papular erythemic lesions inside striae distensae

[99]. In one report in 87% of cases the lesions began at the umbilicus [45]. The other half begin with typical lesions, but in an atypical distribution (onset on the extremities or the palms and soles) [99]. A mild case may show only a few scattered papules or a few erythematous plaques of small diameter [91].

Fig. 12.7 Herpes gestationis. Bullous lesions

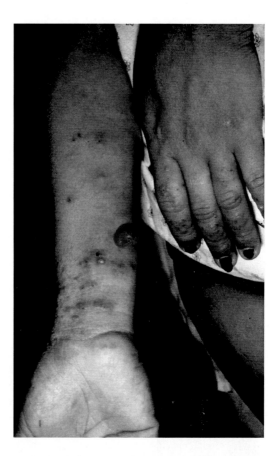

Fig. 12.8 Herpes gestationis. On soles (test for fungus was negative and patch tests showed negative reactions)

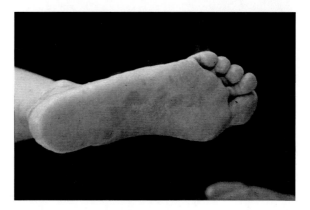

In more severe cases, small vesicles arise in a herpetiform or circinate pattern, frequently coalescing, forming tense bullae. They tend to appear within the margins of the areas of erythematous, urticarial looking bases or adjacent to them [35, 36, 91, 112], although bullae may appear on otherwise clinically uninvolved skin [35].

The bullae are found most frequently on the abdomen, forearms, back, genitalia, and buttocks, but may arise on all body surfaces [36, 91, 112, 113]. By coalescing, they tend to form bizarre geographic patterns extending considerably so that only a few areas are spared [91]. In some cases target lesions are seen [113]. The interval between the onset of the eruption and the development of bullous lesions was found to be usually within 2–4 weeks [45]. The duration of individual lesions is in general 1–3 weeks [78].

As the bullae rupture and dry out, the bare areas become covered with brownish-yellow or hemorrhagic crusts [36, 91]. If secondary infection supervenes, they become purulent and sometimes deeply ulcerated [91]. Usually, however, they heal without scarring [91]. Significant postinflammatory hyperpigmentation may occur [38].

Mucous membrane involvement is not common [113], but lesions of the oral mucosa have been reported in up to about 20% of patients [36]. The face was found to be involved in less than 10% of cases [35, 45]. The eruption may be worsened by bromides and iodides [36].

12.5
Differential Diagnosis

HG can be easily differentiated from the other dermatoses of pregnancy as it is the only condition which produces blisters when the disease is fully developed [113], but nonclassic presentations or the early urticarial papules and plaques may resemble allergic contact dermatitis or pruritic urticarial papules and plaques of pregnancy (PUPPP) [90], and indeed PUPPP is the disease most often mistaken for HG [95]; however, a characteristic structure and direct immunofluorescence will be present even in early lesions of HG [35, 113]. PUPPP rarely appears within the umbilicus, which is a common site for HG. In addition, PUPPP usually occurs in the third trimester and is characterized by the development of urticarial lesions in the striae [90]. Bullae formation is rare in PUPPP, and immunofluorescence testing is negative [90].

Major differential diagnoses include diseases that only accidentally occur in pregnancy [113]. It looks a lot like dermatitis herpetiformis both clinically and histologically [36]. They are both widespread, pruritic, polymorphous bullous eruptions [36]. Histologically, they both display subepidermal bullae and moderate numbers of neutrophils and eosinophils in the bullous fluid and in the dermal infiltrate [36]. They are both frequently associated with a peripheral blood eosinophilia and an increase in urinary chorionic gonadotropin levels [36, 112]. However, the lesion of dermatitis herpetiformis is that of clusters of vesicles and not bullae without plaque formation [19]. Treatment of dermatitis herpetiformis includes sulfonamides (sulfapyridine) because corticosteroids have little or no success [19].

Other differential diagnoses include erythema multiforme, pemphigus vulgaris, pemphigus foliaceus, and bullous drug reactions [112]. These entities are differentiated on histologic or immunologic grounds [113]. Pemphigus vulgaris can be differentiated by its flaccid bullae arising from normal-appearing skin [19]. Histologic examination shows acantholytic cells within the blisters [19]. Impetigo herpetiformis is different in that pustules arise from an erythematous base, and fever and hypocalcemia are often present [19].

12.6
Relationship Between Herpes Gestationis and Bullous Pemphigoid

As described in Sect. 12.2, there are many similarities noted between HG and BP. The similarities are not only clinical (even more than dermatitis herpetiformis in that plaques of redness and swelling are associated with the bullae), but also histopathologic and immunopathologic [14, 42, 74]. These similarities led Holmes and Black [41] in 1982 to suggest that "herpes gestationis" should be referred to as "pemphigoid gestationis." However, it should be emphasized that although HG has many similarities to BP, which justify its inclusion within the pemphigoid group of disorders, it is nevertheless a distinct disorder [42].

The similarities and differences between these two disorders are summarized in Box 12.1.

Box 12.1 Summary of the similarities and differences between herpes gestationis (HG) and bullous pemphigoid (BP) [1, 5, 12, 14, 20, 32, 34, 40–42, 45, 47, 53, 54, 79, 96, 102]

Similarities between HG and BP

> *Clinical appearance* – both present as pruritic urticarial lesions which develop into large, tense bullae
> *Treatment response* – both highly responsive to steroid treatment
> *Histopathology* – both demonstrate subepidermal bullae containing numerous eosinophils; ultrastructural studies show that in both there is a linear deposition of IgG within the lamina lucida
> *Physiopathology* – the diseases share a common antigen that is targeted by antibodies – BPAG1 (230-kDa protein) and BPAG2 (180-kDa protein)
> *Autoimmune association* – both were described in association with several autoantibody-related diseases

Differences between HG and BP

> *Onset of disease* – HG occurs in women of childbearing age; BP is a disease of children and the elderly
> *Clinical appearance* – presence of umbilical lesions in HG (not apparent in BP)
> *Triggers for disease* – HG is associated with pregnancy, menstruation, and steroid hormones; BP has no known initiators
> *Antibody characteristics* – low antibody titer in conventional immunofluorescence tests and avid complement fixation in HG; increased antibody titer and decreased ability to fix complement in BP
> *Histopathology* – electron microscopy revealed necrotic keratinocytes at the dermoepidermal junction, which are rare in BP but a regular feature of HG
> *Immunogenetics* – in HG there is a significantly increased frequency of human leukocyte antigen (HLA)-DR3 and HLA-DR4; in BP the frequencies of HLAs are normal.

12

12.7
Laboratory Findings

Direct immunofluorescence offers the most useful information for diagnosis [24, 38]. To obtain a diagnostic punch biopsy, it is recommended that the biopsy site be at the normal-appearing perilesional skin to prevent artifacts produced by tissue necrosis within lesions [114].

Immunofluorescence examination of patients with HG revealed a bandlike deposit of C3 as a constant finding, often associated with C1q, C4, C5, factor B, and properdin within the basement membrane zone (BMZ) between the epidermis and the dermis [10, 59, 64, 78, 85] (Fig. 12.9).

IgG deposits have also been reported to be present in the skin of 25–50% of patients with HG at the BMZ; however, studies with monoclonal antibodies showed IgG1 deposition in the BMZ of skin in all patients [2]. IgA and IgM deposits are seen much less often [24, 45, 64, 68, 91]. In salt split skin specimens, antibody deposition is found along the base of the epidermal section, similar to the staining outline seen in BP [80]. Occasionally, staining may be seen along both the epidermal and the dermal sections [80]. Linear deposition of IgG1 and C3 has also been shown among the BMZ of amniotic epithelium, as well as in the skin of neonates of affected mothers [63, 77]. The immunoreactants may persist for more than 1 year after the lesions have cleared [78].

A circulating, complement-binding factor (the "HG factor") was found in most cases in the sera of patients with HG in 1976 [59, 91]. Although long thought not to be an immunoglobulin, because it was primarily mistakenly thought to be heat-labile [85], this HG factor was later characterized by Katz to be an IgG type of BMZ antibody which activates in vivo the classic and alternate pathway of complement [55, 59]. Instead of the regular indirect immunofluorescence, complement indirect immunoflu-

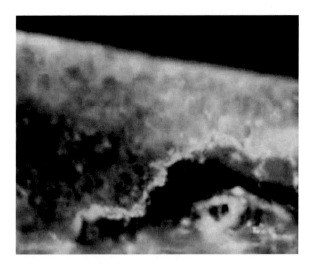

Fig. 12.9 Herpes gestationis. Direct immunofluorescence: linear deposition of C3 at the dermoepidermal junction

orescence must be used [113]. In this technique, normal tissue substrate is incubated with patient serum that has been heated to destroy any complement-fixing activity [113]. HG factor binds to the substrate during incubation [113]. When a source of complement (e.g., human serum) is added, HG factor activates many molecules of C3 which bind to the substrate along the BMZ [113]. Incubation with fluorescein-labeled antihuman C3 antibodies will then stain the C3 molecules so that they can be observed with fluorescence microscopy [113]. Anti-BMZ antibody titers do not correlate with the extent or severity of the disease [102].

An increased incidence of antigastric parietal cell antibodies has been reported [100], and increased antithyroid antibody titers have been documented [45, 100], but clinically apparent thyroid dysfunction has rarely been reported [99]. Antinuclear antigens and complement levels are normal [99].

In addition to the immunologic findings, peripheral leukocytosis with an eosinophilia of 10–50% has been observed [68, 113]. Eosinophilia has been said to correlate with the severity of the disease [68], but this observation has not been verified [99]. There might also be en elevated sedimentation rate and increased urinary chorionic gonadotropin levels [109].

12.8
Histopathology

The early-stage urticarial, nonblistered areas show nonspecific findings of superficial and deep, dense, perivascular infiltrate of lymphocytes, histiocytes, and eosinophils, often characterized as a "reactive privasculitis" [11, 38]. Spongiosis and vacuolization of epidermal cells, at times severe enough to form intraepidermal microvesicles, may be seen [115] (Fig. 12.9). Eosinophils may be found in the spongiotic foci within the epidermis [38] (Figs. 12.10, 12.11).

There is marked dermal edema, spongiosis, and necrosis of basal cells at the tip of the dermal papillae [38]. The dermal infiltrate may vary from almost completely lymphocytic with few eosinophils to predominantly eosinophilic with nuclear fragmentation (nuclear dust) [115]. These features may sometimes be indistinguishable from erythema multiforme in the former case, or BP or dermatitis herpetiformis in the latter case [36, 91].

As the condition develops, bullae shaped like an inverted teardrop arise at the dermoepidermal junction, containing neutrophils and eosinophils [11, 91, 95]. The degree of edema and vesiculation is varable [35].

Ultrastructural studies demonstrate that the earliest modification is damage mainly to the basal cell plasma membrane, leading to destruction of basal cells with blister formation, while the basement membrane remains on the floor of the bulla [115]. Ultimately the basement membrane is also disrupted [115]. Necrosis may be seen not only of basal cells but of squamous cells as well [24]. Ultrastructurally the level of splitting occurs in the lamina lucida [35].

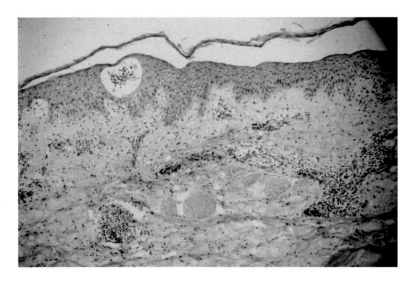

Fig. 12.10 Herpes gestationis. Hematoxylin and eosin stain. Intra- and subepidermal vesicles, dermal edema, lymphocytic infiltration, eosinophils, basal cell necrosis

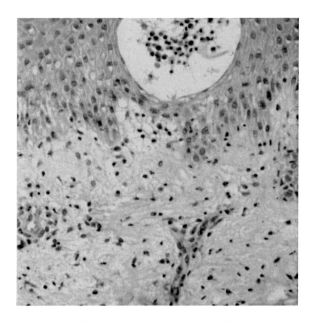

Fig. 12.11 Herpes gestationis. Hematoxylin and eosin stain. Close view. Note numerous eosinophils, basal cell necrosis

12.9
Physiopathology

The cause of the disease was debated for many years. It was first believed to be an allergic reaction to the products of conception [19]. Later, many specific causes were suggested, including toxic effects of fetal and placental tissues, infectious agents, impaired renal and hepatic function, ovarian hypofunction, increased production of chorionic gonadotropin, and Rh isosensitization [112, 113]. However, through use of ultrastructural and immuno-logic methods, and based on the mode of presentation, HG is now regarded by most as a specific entity within the group of autoimmune diseases [91].

The autoantibody or HG factor is derived from a subclass of IgG (IgG1) having a very strong complement-activation ability [91]. The in vivo binding of early complement components nec-essary for the activation of both the classic (C1q, C4) and alternate (properdin) complement pathways implicates both routes in the deposition of C3 at the BMZ, along the upper part of the lumina lucida [33, 58, 59]. Chemoattraction of eosinophils and their subsequent degranulation follow [99]. It is presumably the release of proteolytic enzymes from eosinophilic granules that dissolves the bond between epidermis and dermis, forming bullae [96, 99].

The antigen against which the HG factor is directed was found by immunoblotting to be a 180-kDa glycoprotein, identified as the BP antigen 2 (BPAG2, also called type XVII collagen) [7, 63, 77]. The antigen itself is not abnormal, because it is a normal skin constituent [96]. Instead, it is the actual creation of antibodies against the antigen that is pathologic [98]. Epitope mapping has demonstrated that HG autoantibodies bind a common antigenic site within the noncollagneous domain (NC16A) of the antigen (epitopes A1, A2, A.25, and A3) [29, 57, 72].

Much work has been done to describe BPAG2 [99]. This autoantigen is a transmem-brane collagenous protein. Its amino-terminal end is fixed within the intracellular com-ponent of the hemidesmosome, and its carboxy-terminal end is positioned extracellularly, between the plasma membrane of the basal keratincoyte and the lamina lucida [28, 29]. It may function as a cell matrix protein that mediates connection of hemidesmosomes to the underlying BMZ [28, 70]. With use of molecular genetic studies the BP antigen gene has been localized to the long arm of chromosome 10 [70]. It is a gene product different from another hemidesmosomal protein, the BP antigen 1, a 230-kDa intracellular protein that corresponds to the major autoantigen of BP [6, 63, 77]. This latter antigen may also be recognized by some HG sera [63].

Antibody titers and direct immunofluorescence tests for C3 may remain positive even after clearance of the skin lesions, raising speculation that factors other than an antibody to BPAG2 may contribute to blister formation in HG [92].

There is a strong predisposition for the development of HG in studies of HLA [35]. It has been noted that there is a high frequency of HLA-B8, HLA-DR3, and HLA-DR4 [45]. HLA-DR3 alone was seen in 61–80% of patients, as opposed to 22% in the normal population, 52–53% have HLA-DR4, and 43–50% have the combination of both HLA-DR3 and HLA-DR4 [45, 102]. Only 3% of normal women share this antigen grouping [102]. It is interesting to note that according to one calculation, if 3% of normal women have the HLA-DR3–HLA-DR4 combination and only one in 50,000 women develop HG, then less than 1% of women with the predisposing antigen combination actually develop it

[97]. HLA-DR3 shows linkage disequilibrium with the C4 null allele, and a corresponding increase in the level of the C4 null allele has been reported [108]. This disequilibrium may be important by leading to impaired immune complex degradation [2].

It is not understood how these antigens contribute to the development of HG, as some patients do not express either antigen, which suggests that the cause of HG is probably multifactorial, as genetic (HLA-type) and environmental (pregnancy) factors contribute to its pathogenesis [2].

It is well known that patients with autoimmune diseases and their family members are more susceptible to the development of other autoimmune diseases or the production of autoantibodies [2]. Graves's disease, autoimmune thyroiditis, type I diabetes, idiopathic Addison's disease, chronic active hepatitis, celiac disease, dermatitis herpetiformis, suba-cute cutaneous lupus erythematosus, dermatomyositis, scleroderma, and Sjogren's disease also have HLA-DR3 and HLA-DR4 as a major component of their pathogenesis [35]. In accordance with these facts, the coexistence of HG and other autoimmune diseases such as Graves's disease, Hashimoto's thyroiditis, alopecia areata, ulcerative colitis, vitiligo, and pernicious anemia has been observed [35, 90, 100]. Graves's disease subsequently develops in 11% of patients with HG (compared with only a 0.4% incidence in the nor-mal female population) [100, 101]. There is also a slight increase in the levels of other autoantibodies, including antithyroid antibodies and gastric parietal cell antibodies [100]. Incidents of autoimmune diseases are higher (25%) in relatives of patients with HG, com-monly Graves's disease, but also Hashimoto's thyroiditis and pernicious anemia [2, 95].

The existence of HLA-DR3 has been related to an impaired ability to clear immune complexes from the serum [69]. An unsophisticated explanation for the HLA association in HG is that it is one of many diseases that tend to take place with HLA-DR3 or HLA-DR4 on the basis of a nonspecific but increased immune response or decreased ability to clear antigen–antibody complexes [35].

What initiates the production of autoantibodies remains unsolved, but because HG is exclusively a disease of pregnancy (or trophoblastic tumors), attention has focused on immu-nogenetics and the potential for cross-reactivity between placental tissues and skin [99].

Unique to the initial development of HG is the presence of placental tissue and the allogenic state of pregnancy [35]. The HG antibody binds to amniotic basement membrane [62, 81], which is derived from fetal ectoderm and is antigenically similar to skin, with both pemphigoid and pemphigus antigens represented [87]. Women with HG also show an increase in the levels of major histocompatibility class II antigens (DR, DP, DQ) within the villous stroma of chorionic villi, adjacent to the maternal decidua, together with an increased number of lymphocytes near the site of immune attack [7, 61]. Therefore, it has been pro-posed that HG is a disease initiated by the aberrant expression of major histocompatibility class II antigens (of paternal haplotype) during the second trimester [60]. This may result in the formation of autoantibodies against a placental antigen that cross-react with a normal basement membrane component of the skin, the 180-kDa BP antigen 2 [3, 7, 60].

In support of the placental-involvement theory is the fact that HG has been reported in association with choriocarcinomas in women, but not in men. In women, the origin of nonovarian choriocarcinoma is placental, involving genetic material from both the patient and the companion; in men, the derivation of choriocarcinoma is syngeneic. Therefore, it seems that placental tissue is a precondition to initiate HG, suggesting a paternal contribu-tion to the development of disease [97].

As exciting as this model is, it has been proved false [96]. Shornick [97] demonstrated that not only does antibody eluted from HG placental basement membrane not bind to the skin, but also that HG serum is unable to fix complement to normal basement membrane or to HG placental tissue. Thus, the elucidation of the role of the placenta in HG initiation will require more work.

Other possibilities for the exact role placental tissue might play in the induction of HG might include modifications in immune regulation secondary to reactions to other placenta antigens, changes in antigen or antibody metabolism or regulation induced by placental hormones, or emission of an as yet unidentified distinctive placental product [97].

Anti-HLA antibodies were found in 85–100% of HG cases, compared with 25% of normal multiparous controls [86, 103, 106, 107]. Because the only source of dissimilar HLAs is characteristically the placenta (which is above all of paternal origin), the widespread finding of anti-HLA antibodies implies a high frequency of immunologic insult during gestation [99]. However, they do not appear to play a direct role in the activation of complement, and how these antibodies relate to the development of HG remains to be determined [86, 99, 103, 106]. It appears that anti-HLA antibodies are an epiphenomenon in the disease process and do not contribute to its pathogenesis [23].

Since the disease flares with pregnancy, menstruation, and oral contraceptive use, it seems likely that female sex hormones may trigger the production of autoantibodies [91]. Despite numerous "clues," the precise nature of the hormonal control remains obscure and it has not been possible so far to utilize it in the management of the disease [41]. One possible explanation might be that estrogens exert their effects by increasing antibody production or altering the effector pathway mechanisms [35].

12.10
Treatment

Therapy is directed at controlling symptoms (mainly to alleviate pruritus) and cutaneous disease (prevent new blister formation) [2, 78]. Treatment of HG depends on the severity of the accompanying pruritus [11]. Mild cases (before the vesiculobullous stage) can be managed with application of potent topical fluorinated corticosteroid creams and lotions, and topical or systemic antihistamines [2, 25, 91, 95]; however, these topical applications are usually ineffective in HG [99]. Patients should be reassured and told that the disease is expected to clear after delivery [91].

More severely affected patients can usually be controlled only by systemic steroids [74], the cornerstone of therapy, usually required when the eruption reaches it bullous stage [45, 99]. A varying daily dosage of between 15 and 40 mg prednisolone in divided doses is usually satisfactory [19, 45]. Dosages higher than 80 mg daily are exceptional [35], although dosages up to 180 mg daily have been used [68]. Individual therapy is adjusted according to the patient's clinical course, as patients are followed closely throughout the pregnancy [78]. Lesions will clear after a few days of treatment and the dose of prednisone should then (after 7–10 days) be reduced to the minimum that will keep the disease under control [91, 96]. Tapered discontinuation should be attempted only in the postpartum period, and the dose should be tapered within days or weeks depending on the clinical response

[2, 91]. A rapid increase in the prednisolone therapy will probably be required immediately postpartum to cover the clinical exacerbation that occurs at this time [42].

Several other agents have been used in those few patients who are refractory to corticosteroids [36]. The most difficult cases may require the addition of azathioprine to the regimen [113]. Some patients respond to pyridoxine hydrochloride (vitamin B_6) in pharmacologic dosages of 400 mg daily [9, 36, 74]. Sulfones and sulfapyridine may control the eruption, but are less effective than in dermatitis herpetiformis [36]. Other drugs with a pyridine nucleus may be effective, including 50 mg pyribenzamine four times daily, and 200–400 mg niacin daily [36]. Some patients unresponsive to steroids were treated and responded to dapsone (Avlosulfon) in the past [11, 113]. However, nowadays dapsone is contraindicated because it was found to be ineffective and can cause hemolytic disease in the newborn [50, 95, 97]. Pulsed-dose intravenously administered cyclophosphamide and cyclosporine have also shown benefits in some patients [15, 82].

Several other adjuvants to corticosteroids (gold, methotrexate) have been tried [99], but none are useful before term, and the experience with each has been variable at best [99]. Ritodrine, a β-agonist used for the treatment of premature labor, was successful in one patient [73]. High-dose intravenously administered immunoglobulin in combination with cyclosporine has also been used [37].

Plasmapheresis has been used successfully in HG in the postpartum period and also during pregnancy itself [14, 111], but its use is limited by logistics and expense [97]. It may be considered in severe and recalcitrant cases [95].

A reversible chemical oophorectomy using luteinizing hormone-releasing hormone analogues (goserelin) produced a remission in a patient with severe HG requiring high doses of oral steroids [27]. Case reports indicate some benefit from tetracyclines in postpartum HG [92]. Finally, early delivery may be required in intractable cases [66].

It should be noted that one should always consider the risk for the patient and the fetus when using a more aggressive treatment, as the rash and accompanying symptoms in almost 100% of patients subside after delivery.

12.11
Prognosis

HG rarely causes serious maternal complications [11]; therefore, it is important not to create significant risk from therapy [99]. Maternal morbidity corresponds to the severity of HG, its duration, and its intrinsic rate of complications, which are usually infectious [91], but this disorder may produce occasional albuminuria and edema [36]. Steroid therapy efficiently suppresses this morbidity, but may add its own unwanted side effects [91]. Because of estrogen-induced flare-ups, patients should consider nonhormonal contraceptive methods [91]. Following the use of systemic antibiotics and steroids, maternal mortality from sepsis is now a rarity [91]. Those with a history of HG seem to be at increased risk for the development of Graves's disease [45, 100].

The prognosis for the infant has been debated for many years [65]. Some investigators reported increased fetal mortality, with association of up to 50% of these pregnancies with fetal complications, including miscarriage, stillbirth, and congenital anomalies [16, 36, 89]. In a literature review of 40 cases, Lawley et al. [68], who added immunologic criteria to patient selection, reported in 1978 23% prematurity (compared with 5% in the general population) and 7.7% stillbirth (compared with 1.3%). One case of fetal cerebral hemorrhage was reported [84]. However, data collected from reported patients tend to be biased toward cases with a more severe outcome [42].

Others report that the condition does not appear to carry any risk to the fetus [42, 65]. A literature review by Kolodny [65] in 1969 concluded that there was no increase in stillbirth or abortion associated with HG. Shornick et al. [104] in 1983 reported 28 patients and 102 pregnancies with no increased risk of prematurity or spontaneous abortion. In the study by Holmes et al. [45] of 24 patients with 39 pregnancies affected by HG, there were no stillbirths or neonatal deaths. The average birth weight was 2.86 kg, and the average gestation was 39 weeks [45]. Holmes and Black [42] feel that fetal prognosis in HG has probably been beneficially affected by the advent of corticosteroid therapy [42].

In a referral setting in 1984, Holmes and Black [43] reported a significant increase in small-for-gestational age (SGA) infants in 33 patients with HG and 50 pregnancies that progressed to delivery. They advised patients with HG to plan for delivery in units with facilities for intensive care of the newborn because of increased risk of fetal complications in infants of low gestational weight [43]. In 1992, a study by Shornick and Black [101] involving 74 patients and 254 pregnancies was published, and included 24 pregnancies from the study by Holmes et al. [45]. They found a minor propensity toward SGA babies and an increased frequency of prematurity [101]. Sixteen percent of deliveries associated with HG occurred before 36 weeks, and 32% occurred before 38 weeks, compared with 2 and 11%, respectively, in the same women during unaffected pregnancies [101].

Since pemphigoid gestationis affects not only the skin but also the placenta, clinical evidence of placental insufficiency, such as low birth weight and prematurity, is not an unexpected finding [101].

Because of the question of an increased risk of prematurity and SGA and the hypothesis that underlying placental insufficiency may be the cause, once the diagnosis of HG has been established the pregnancy should be considered to be high risk [23, 43]. Fetal surveillance in the third trimester of pregnancy is warranted [43, 100]. A modified biophysical profile (nonstress test and amniotic fluid volume) on a weekly basis should be sufficient unless evidence exists for growth restriction [96]. More frequent testing would then be indicated, including Doppler flow studies of the umbilical arteries [96].

Cutaneous involvement of the newborn of an affected mother occurs in 5–10% of cases [18, 35]. Of the 36 infants born to mothers with HG, Lawley et al. [68] found four with lesions resembling HG. Two of these infants had circulating HG factors in their blood, two of the infants had complement detected in their skin by direct immunofluorescence, and one had circulating anti-BMZ antibody of the IgG class [68]. This highly suggests passive placental transfer of the disease and a pathogenic role for the HG factor [17, 91]. Positive immunofluorescence tests from newborn skin biopsy specimens, in the absence of clinically apparent disease, have been demonstrated repeatedly [97]. Subclinical disease is probably common, despite the absence of clinical disease [2]. The lesions may become superinfected as the immune system of the neonate is not fully developed [67].

12

Summary

> Herpes gestationis (HG) is a hormonally mediated autoimmune bullous disorder of pregnancy.
> The incidence varies considerably, probably between 1:50,000 and 1:60,000.
> Onset is usually during the second trimester, but it can present in any phase of pregnancy or the puerperium.
> Recurrences are common in subsequent pregnancies, with oral contraceptive use, and before menstruation.
> It presents first as pruritic erythematous plaques which later form vesicles and bullae.
> Direct immunofluorescence is diagnostic, revealing deposition of C3 at the basement membrane zone (BMZ) in all cases. HG factor may be found in the blood.
> The HG factor is directed against BPAG2, leading to complement activation and destruction of the BMZ. HLA-DR3 and HLA-DR4 were fond to be associated with the disease.
> Mild cases can be controlled with topical steroids. Bullous disease will probably necessitate systemic corticosteroids.
> Complications for the mother are rare. Fetal prognosis is debatable, but presumably there is no increased risk for fetal death. SGA babies and prematurity may be seen owing to placental insufficiency. The pregnancy should be considered high risk with strict fetal surveillance during the third trimester.

References

1. Ahmed AR, Cohen E, Blumenson LE et al (1977) HLA in bullous pemphigoid. Arch Dermatol 113:1121
2. Al-Fares SI, Jones SV, Black MM (2001) The specific dermatoses of pregnancy: a re-appraisal. J Eur Acad Dermatol Venereol 15:197–206
3. Black M, Stephens C (1989) The specific dermatoses of pregnancy: the British perspective. Adv Dermatol 7:105–127
4. Black MM (1997) Progress and new directions in the investigation of the specific dermatoses of pregnancy. Keio J Med 46:40–41
5. Bor S, Feiwel M, Chanarin I (1969) Vitiligo and its aetiological relationship to organ-specific autoimmune disease. Br J Dermatol 81:83–88
6. Borradori L, Saurat JH (1994) Specific dermatoses of pregnancy. Toward a comprehensive view? Arch Dermatol 130:778–780
7. Borthwick GM, Holmes RC, Stirrat GM (1988) Abnormal expression of class II MHC antigens in placentae from patients with pemphigoid gestationis: analysis of class II MHC subregion product expression. Placenta 9:81–94
8. Bunel J (1811) Essai sur le pemphugus. Paris
9. Burkhart CG (1982) Pyridoxine-responsive herpes gestationis. Arch Dermatol 118:535
10. Bushkell LL, Jordon RE, Goltz RW (1974) Herpes gestationis. New immunologic findings. Arch Dermatol 110:65–69

11. Callen JP (1984) Pregnancy's effects on the skin. Common and uncommon changes. Postgrad Med 75:138–145

12. Callen JP, Anderson TF, Chanda JJ et al (1978) Bullous pemphigoid and other disorders associated with autoimmune phenomena. Arch Dermatol 114:245–246

13. Carruthers JA (1978) Herpes gestationis: a reappraisal. Clin Exp Dermatol 3:199–202

14. Carruthers JA, Black MM, Ramnarain N (1977) Immunopathological studies in herpes gestationis. Br J Dermatol 96:35–43

15. Castle SP, Mather-Mondrey M, Bennion S et al (1996) Chronic herpes gestationis and antiphospholipid antibody syndrome successfully treated with cyclophosphamide. J Am Acad Dermatol 34:333–336

16. Cawley EP, Wheeler CE, Wilhite PA (1952) Herpes gestationis and the Rh factor. South Med J 45:827–832

17. Chorzelski TP, Jablonska S, Beutner EH et al (1976) Herpes gestations with identical lesions in the newborn. Passive transfer of the disease? Arch Dermatol 112:1129–1131

18. Cohen LM (1998) Dermatoses of pregnancy. West J Med 169:223–224

19. Dacus JV (1990) Pruritus in pregnancy. Clin Obstet Gynecol 33:738–745

20. Doniach D, Roitt IM, Taylor KB (1965) Autoimmunity in pernicious anemia and thyroiditis: a family study. Ann N Y Acad Sci 124:605–625

21. Duhring L (1885) Med News 47:421

22. Dupont C (1974) Herpes gestationis with hydatidiform mole. Trans St Johns Hosp Dermatol Soc 60:103

23. Engineer L, Bhol K, Ahmed AR (2000) Pemphigoid gestationis: a review. Am J Obstet Gynecol 183:483–491

24. Eudy SF, Baker GF (1990) Dermatopathology for the obstetrician. Clin Obstet Gynecol 33:728–737

25. Flowers FP, Sherertz EF (1985) Immunologic disorders of the skin and mucous membranes. Med Clin North Am 69:657–673

26. Garcia-Gonzalez E, Castro-Llamas J, Karchmer S et al (1999) Class II major histocompatibility complex typing across the ethnic barrier in pemphigoid gestationis. A study in Mexicans. Int J Dermatol 38:46–51

27. Garvey MP, Handfield-Jones SE, Black MM (1992) Pemphigoid gestationis – response to chemical oophorectomy with goserelin. Clin Exp Dermatol 17:443–445

28. Giudice GJ, Emery DJ, Diaz LA (1992) Cloning and primary structural analysis of the bullous pemphigoid autoantigen BP180. J Invest Dermatol 99:243–250

29. Giudice GJ, Emery DJ, Zelickson BD et al (1993) Bullous pemphigoid and herpes gestationis autoantibodies recognize a common non-collagenous site on the BP180 ectodomain. J Immunol 151:5742–5750

30. Goodall J (1988) Routine immunofluorescence for pruritic urticarial papules and plaques of pregnancy. J Am Acad Dermatol 18:1146

31. Goodall J (1990) Immunofluorescence biopsy for pruritic urticarial papules and plaques of pregnancy. J Am Acad Dermatol 22:322

32. Hamilton DV, McKenzie AW (1978) Bullous pemphigoid and primary biliary cirrhosis. Br J Dermatol 99:447–450

33. Harrington CI, Bleehen SS (1979) Herpes gestationis: immunopathological and ultrastructural studies. Br J Dermatol 100:389–399

34. Hashimoto K, Miki Y, Nakata S et al (1979) HLA antigens in bullous pemphigoid among Japanese. Arch Dermatol 115:96–97

35. Hayashi RH (1990) Bullous dermatoses and prurigo of pregnancy. Clin Obstet Gynecol 33:746–753

36. Hellreich P (1974) The skin changes of pregnancy. Cutis 13:82–86

37. Hern S, Harman K, Bhogal BS et al (1998) A severe persistent case of pemphigoid gestationis treated with intravenous immunoglobulins and cyclosporin. Clin Exp Dermatol 23:185–188
38. Hertz KC, Katz SI, Maize J et al (1976) Herpes gestationis. A clinicopathologic study. Arch Dermatol 112:1543–1548
39. Holmes R, Black M (1983) Herpes gestationis. Dermatol Clin 1:195
40. Holmes RC, Black MM (1980) Herpes gestationis. A possible association with autoimmune thyrotoxicosis (Graves' disease). J Am Acad Dermatol 3:474–477
41. Holmes RC, Black MM (1982) The specific dermatoses of pregnancy: a reappraisal with special emphasis on a proposed simplified clinical classification. Clin Exp Dermatol 7:65–73
42. Holmes RC, Black MM (1983) The specific dermatoses of pregnancy. J Am Acad Dermatol 8:405–412
43. Holmes RC, Black MM (1984) The fetal prognosis in pemphigoid gestationis (herpes gestationis). Br J Dermatol 110:67–72
44. Holmes RC, Williamson DM, Black MM (1986) Herpes gestationis persisting for 12 years post partum. Arch Dermatol 122:375–376
45. Holmes RC, Black MM, Dann J et al (1982) A comparative study of toxic erythema of pregnancy and herpes gestationis. Br J Dermatol 106:499–510
46. Holmes RC, Black MM, Jurecka W et al (1983) Clues to the aetiology and pathogenesis of herpes gestationis. Br J Dermatol 109:131–139
47. Honigsmann H, Stingl G, Holubar K et al (1976) Herpes gestationis: fine structural pattern of immunoglobulin deposits in the skin in vivo. J Invest Dermatol 66:389–392
48. Ibbotson SH, Lawrence CM (1995) An uninvolved pregnancy in a patient after a previous episode of herpes gestationis. Arch Dermatol 131:1091–1092
49. Jablonska S, Chorzelski TP, Maciejowska E et al (1975) Immunologic phenomena in herpes gestations. Their pathogenic and diagnostic significance. J Dermatol 2:149–158
50. Jenkins R, Shornick J, Black M (1993) Pemphigoid gestationis. J Eur Acad Dermatol Venereol 2:163–173
51. Jenkins RE, Jones SA, Black MM (1996) Conversion of pemphigoid gestationis to bullous pemphigoid – two refractory cases highlighting this association. Br J Dermatol 135:595–598
52. Jenkins RE, Hern S, Black MM (1999) Clinical features and management of 87 patients with pemphigoid gestationis. Clin Exp Dermatol 24:255–259
53. Jordon RE, Nordby JM, Milstein H (1975) The complement system in bullous pemphigoid. III. Fixation of C1q and C4 by pemphigoid antibody. J Lab Clin Med 86:733–740
54. Jordon RE, Muller SA, Hale WL et al (1969) Bullous pemphigoid associated with systemic lupus erythematosus. Arch Dermatol 99:17–25
55. Jordon RE, Heine KG, Tappeiner G et al (1976) The immunopathology of herpes gestationis. Immunofluorescence studies and characterization of "HG factor". J Clin Invest 57:1426–1431
56. Jorgensen EH, Clemmensen O, Anagnostaki L (1987) Herpes gestationis. Acta Obstet Gynecol Scand 66:175–177
57. Karpati S, Stolz W, Meurer M et al (1991) Herpes gestationis: ultrastructural identification of the extracellular antigenic sites in diseased skin using immunogold techniques. Br J Dermatol 125:317–324
58. Katz A, Minto JO, Toole JW et al (1977) Immunopathologic study of herpes gestationis in mother and infant. Arch Dermatol 113:1069–1072
59. Katz SI, Hertz KC, Yaoita H (1976) Herpes gestationis. Immunopathology and characterization of the HG factor. J Clin Invest 57:1434–1441
60. Kelly SE, Black MM, Fleming S (1989) Pemphigoid gestationis: a unique mechanism of initiation of an autoimmune response by MHC class II molecules? J Pathol 158:81–82

61. Kelly SE, Black MM, Fleming S (1990) Antigen-presenting cells in the skin and placenta in pemphigoid gestationis. Br J Dermatol 122:593–599
62. Kelly SE, Bhogal BS, Wojnarowska F et al (1988) Expression of a pemphigoid gestationis-related antigen by human placenta. Br J Dermatol 118:605–611
63. Kelly SE, Bhogal BS, Wojnarowska F et al (1990) Western blot analysis of the antigen in pemphigoid gestationis. Br J Dermatol 122:445–449
64. Kocsis M, Eeg TL, Husby G et al (1975) Immunofluorescence studies in herpes gestationis. Acta Derm Venereol 55:25–29
65. Kolodny RC (1969) Herpes gestationis. A new assessment of incidence, diagnosis, and fetal prognosis. Am J Obstet Gynecol 104:39–45
66. Kroumpouzos G, Cohen LM (2001) Dermatoses of pregnancy. J Am Acad Dermatol 45:1–19; quiz 19–22
67. Kroumpouzos G, Cohen LM (2003) Specific dermatoses of pregnancy: an evidence-based systematic review. Am J Obstet Gynecol 188:1083–1092
68. Lawley TJ, Stingl G, Katz SI (1978) Fetal and maternal risk factors in herpes gestationis. Arch Dermatol 114:552–555
69. Lawley TJ, Hall RP, Fauci AS et al (1981) Defective Fc-receptor functions associated with the HLA-B8/DRw3 haplotype: studies in patients with dermatitis herpetiformis and normal subjects. N Engl J Med 304:185–192
70. Li KH, Sawamura D, Giudice GJ et al (1991) Genomic organization of collagenous domains and chromosomal assignment of human 180-kDa bullous pemphigoid antigen-2, a novel collagen of stratified squamous epithelium. J Biol Chem 266:24064–24069
71. Lim HW, Bystryn JC (1978) Evaluation and management of diseases of the vulva: bullous diseases. Clin Obstet Gynecol 21:1007–1022
72. Lin MS, Gharia M, Fu CL et al (1999) Molecular mapping of the major epitopes of BP180 recognized by herpes gestationis autoantibodies. Clin Immunol 92:285–292
73. Macdonald KJ, Raffle EJ (1984) Ritodrine therapy associated with remission of pemphigoid gestationis. Br J Dermatol 111:630
74. McKenzie AW (1971) Skin disorders in pregnancy. Practitioner 206:773–780
75. Milton J (1872) The pathology and treatment of diseases of the skin. Hardwicke, London
76. Morgan JK (1968) Herpes gestationis influenced by an oral contraceptive. Br J Dermatol 80:456–458
77. Morrison LH, Labib RS, Zone JJ et al (1988) Herpes gestationis autoantibodies recognize a 180-kD human epidermal antigen. J Clin Invest 81:2023–2026
78. Murray JC (1990) Pregnancy and the skin. Dermatol Clin 8:327–334
79. Obasi OE, Savin JA (1977) Pemphigoid and pernicious anaemia. Br Med J 2:1458–1459
80. Onodera Y, Shimizu H, Hashimoto T et al (1994) Difference in binding sites of autoantibodies against 230- and 170-kD bullous pemphigoid antigens on salt-split skin. J Invest Dermatol 102:686–690
81. Ortonne JP, Hsi BL, Verrando P et al (1987) Herpes gestationis factor reacts with the amniotic epithelial basement membrane. Br J Dermatol 117:147–154
82. Paternoster DM, Bruno G, Grella PV (1997) New observations on herpes gestationis therapy. Int J Gynaecol Obstet 56:277–278
83. Pierard J, Thiery M, Kint A (1969) Histology and ultrastructure of herpes gestationis. Arch Belg Dermatol Syphiligr 25:321–335
84. Powell J, Wojnarowska F, James M et al (2000) Pemphigoid gestationis with intra-uterine death associated with foetal cerebral haemorrhage in the mid-trimester. Clin Exp Dermatol 25:452–453

85. Provost TT, Tomasi TB Jr (1973) Evidence for complement activation via the alternate pathway in skin diseases, I. Herpes gestationis, systemic lupus erythematosus, and bullous pemphigoid. J Clin Invest 52:1779–1787
86. Reunala T, Karvonen J, Tiilikainen A et al (1977) Herpes gestationis. A high titre of anti-HLA-B8 antibody in the mother and pemphigoid-like immunohistological findings in the mother and the child. Br J Dermatol 96:563–568
87. Robinson HN, Anhalt GJ, Patel HP et al (1984) Pemphigus and pemphigoid antigens are expressed in human amnion epithelium. J Invest Dermatol 83:234–237
88. Roger D, Vaillant L, Fignon A et al (1994) Specific pruritic diseases of pregnancy. A prospective study of 3192 pregnant women. Arch Dermatol 130:734–739
89. Russell B, Thorne NA (1957) Herpes gestationis. Br J Dermatol 69:339–357
90. Rye B, Webb JM (1997) Autoimmune bullous diseases. Am Fam Physician 55:2709–2718
91. Sasseville D, Wilkinson RD, Schnader JY (1981) Dermatoses of pregnancy. Int J Dermatol 20:223–241
92. Satoh S, Seishima M, Sawada Y et al (1999) The time course of the change in antibody titres in herpes gestationis. Br J Dermatol 140:119–123
93. Saurat JH (1989) Immunofluorescence biopsy for pruritic urticarial papules and plaques of pregnancy. J Am Acad Dermatol 20:711
94. Schaumburg-Lever G, Saffold OE, Orfanos CE et al (1973) Herpes gestationis. Histology and ultrastructure. Arch Dermatol 107:888–892
95. Scott JE, Ahmed AR (1998) The blistering diseases. Med Clin North Am 82:1239–1283
96. Sherard GB 3rd, Atkinson SM Jr (2001) Focus on primary care: pruritic dermatological conditions in pregnancy. Obstet Gynecol Surv 56:427–432
97. Shornick JK (1987) Herpes gestationis. J Am Acad Dermatol 17:539–556
98. Shornick JK (1993) Herpes gestationis. Dermatol Clin 11:527–533
99. Shornick JK (1998) Dermatoses of pregnancy. Semin Cutan Med Surg 17:172–181
100. Shornick JK, Black MM (1992) Secondary autoimmune diseases in herpes gestationis (pemphigoid gestationis). J Am Acad Dermatol 26:563–566
101. Shornick JK, Black MM (1992) Fetal risks in herpes gestationis. J Am Acad Dermatol 26:63–68
102. Shornick JK, Stastny P, Gilliam JN (1981) High frequency of histocompatibility antigens HLA-DR3 and DR4 in herpes gestations. J Clin Invest 68:553–555
103. Shornick JK, Stastny P, Gilliam JN (1983) Paternal histocompatibility (HLA) antigens and maternal anti-HLA antibodies in herpes gestationis. J Invest Dermatol 81:407–409
104. Shornick JK, Bangert JL, Freeman RG et al (1983) Herpes gestationis: clinical and histologic features of twenty-eight cases. J Am Acad Dermatol 8:214–224
105. Shornick JK, Meek TJ, Nesbitt LT Jr et al (1984) Herpes gestationis in blacks. Arch Dermatol 120:511–513
106. Shornick JK, Jenkins RE, Briggs DC et al (1993) Anti-HLA antibodies in pemphigoid gestationis (herpes gestationis). Br J Dermatol 129:257–259
107. Shornick JK, Artlett CM, Jenkins RE et al (1993) Complement polymorphism in herpes gestationis: association with C4 null allele. J Am Acad Dermatol 29:545–549
108. Shornick JK, Jenkins RE, Artlett CM et al (1995) Class II MHC typing in pemphigoid gestationis. Clin Exp Dermatol 20:123–126
109. Sodhi VK, Sausker WF (1988) Dermatoses of pregnancy. Am Fam Physician 37:131–138
110. Tillman WG (1950) Herpes gestationis with hydatidiform mole and chorion epithelioma. Br Med J 1:1471
111. Van de Wiel A, Hart HC, Flinterman J et al (1980) Plasma exchange in herpes gestationis. Br Med J 281:1041–1042

112. Wade TR, Wade SL, Jones HE (1978) Skin changes and diseases associated with pregnancy. Obstet Gynecol 52:233–242
113. Winton GB, Lewis CW (1982) Dermatoses of pregnancy. J Am Acad Dermatol 6:977–998
114. Yancey KB (1990) Herpes gestationis. Dermatol Clin 8:727–735
115. Yaoita H, Gullino M, Katz SI (1976) Herpes gestationis. Ultrastructure and ultrastructural localization of in vivo-bound complement. J Invest Dermatol 66:383–388
116. Zurn A, Celebi CR, Bernard P et al (1992) A prospective immunofluorescence study of 111 cases of pruritic dermatoses of pregnancy: IgM anti-basement membrane zone antibodies as a novel finding. Br J Dermatol 126:474–478

Impetigo Herpetiformis

13

13.1
Definition

Impetigo herpetiformis (IH), also called "generalized pustular psoriasis of pregnancy," is a rare but exceptionally serious generalized primary pustular eruption associated with pregnancy or with hypocalcemic states and which may be a variant of pustular psoriasis as it appears in pregnancy [6, 22].

13.2
Introduction

"Impetigo herpetiformis" is the name given to an eruption resembling pustular psoriasis of von Zumbusch. It may arise suddenly in a patient without previous psoriatic skin disease [27], but most patients have chronic psoriasis or have a family member with psoriasis [9]. Not all women who develop IH will develop psoriasis in the future [1].

It is still controversial whether this disorder is specific to pregnancy or only exacerbated by it [25]. There are data indicating that there is actually no difference between IH and pustular psoriasis of von Zumbusch with relation to sex, age, pregnancy, laboratory findings, histologic features, or response to treatment [7]. It was suggested that the only difference between the two is solely the time of appearance – in the past, pregnant women developing a generalized pustular eruption were diagnosed as suffering from IH, and non-pregnant women were diagnosed as having pustular psoriasis of von Zumbusch [9].

IH was first described by von Hebra in 1872 in five women [14]. When first described, this entity was thought to occur in pregnancy and the early postpartum period only [26]; therefore, the disease was considered a dermatosis of pregnancy [27]. Later it was reported in postmenopausal women, in men, and even in children [26]. However, this very rare and serious disease occurs most often in pregnant women [14, 16, 26]. In a review by Moslein

A. Ingber, *Obstetric Dermatology*,
DOI: 10.1007/978-3-540-88399-9, © Springer-Verlag Berlin Heidelberg 2009

[17] of 113 cases described in the literature from 1921 to 1958, it was found that 54% of cases occurred in pregnant women, 36% in nonpregnant women and 10% in men [14]. von Hebra associated this condition with poor maternal and fetal outcome, since four out of his original five patients died [22]. A high mortality rate (25%) was also found in the review by Moslein [14, 17]. Evidence of hypoparathyroidism and hypocalcemia was frequently found in patients, pregnant or not, and an etiologic role for these conditions has been suggested but not proved [23].

13.3
Incidence

IH is a very rare entity [15, 23], with under 200 cases reported in the literature, and even so some of the reported cases do not fulfill all the criteria for the diagnosis of this entity [11, 20, 27].

13.4
Clinical Presentation

When associated with pregnancy, the onset of IH is acute and may begin at any time during gestation, but usually from late in the first trimester to the end of the third trimester, with a peak incidence during the last 3 months [22, 26]. It will fade away spontaneously between pregnancies, but recurrences are expected with subsequent pregnancies, with the rash recurring earlier and with increased severity in succeeding ones [4, 9, 15]. Worsening of pustular psoriasis just before menstruation and with use of oral contraceptives occurs, so the hormonal changes of pregnancy may relate to the severity of IH [13].

The primary lesion in IH is a sterile pustule [4, 23]. The rash usually starts as irregular erythematous macules and patches or slightly raised scaled plaques distributed symmetrically in the lower abdomen, in the inguinogenital region, and in other intertriginous areas (Figs. 13.1, 13.2). Some common specific primary areas of involvement include the umbilicus, medial thighs, axillae, nape and anterior aspect of the neck, inframammary folds, and gluteal creases. On the margins of these very inflamed erythematous bases arise groups or rings of multiple, distinct pinhead sterile pustules. These pustules are small (usually less than 2 mm in diameter), painful, superficial and have a white or greenish color [3, 8, 9, 13, 14, 22, 26, 27].

Areas of involvement progressively enlarge by peripheral extension of the active pustular margin. The central lesions are quickly broken down and exude, leaving denuded areas or becoming crusted, leaving an impetiginized appearance, from which the disease originally took its name [13, 22, 24]. With time, the eruption becomes confluent, and in severe cases ultimately extends to the trunk and extremities to cover the entire skin surface except for the face, hands, and feet with active pustules and older crusted lesions [22, 26]. In flexural areas, the pustules may coalesce and pile up to form crusted and vegetating brownish-red plaques, or condyloma-like lesions, to some extent suggestive of pemphigus

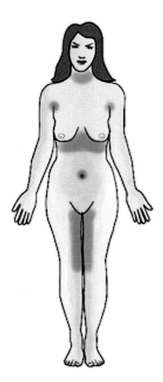 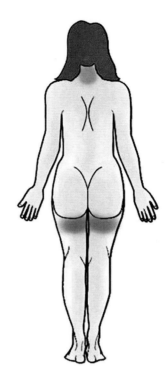

Fig. 13.1 Areas of involvement of impetigo herpetiformis, anterior view

Fig. 13.2 Areas of involvement of impetigo herpetiformis, posterior view

vegetans [14, 22]. The rash may involve mucous membranes such as the tongue, oral buccal mucosa, and esophagus with papules and pustules, leaving painful erosions arranged in a circinate pattern [1, 14, 22, 26]. The oral lesions are painful, grayish-white plaques, resembling the oral lesions seen in pemphigus vulgaris [26]. Bulla formation is exceptional [26]. Subungual pustules may lift the nail plate, resulting in onycholysis or even complete shedding of the nail [22].

Severe systemic symptoms are present in the preponderance of cases [22]. High fever and chills go together with exacerbations of cutaneous lesions [22]. Nausea, vomiting, and diarrhea are not uncommon, with consequential severe dehydration and weight loss [22]. Other constitutional symptoms include pain, tachycardia, malaise, arthritic pains, lymphadenopathy, splenomegaly, and severe prostration [14, 26]. In cases related to hypocalcemia, symptoms of delirium, tetany, and convulsions are more frequent [22]. Pruritus is not a constant symptom with this condition, is usually not a problem [27], and its presence has been variable in some of the reported cases [9].

The course of IH is overall one of continued progression throughout pregnancy [26]; however, it tends to be cyclic, in that periods of active disease interchange with periods of relative quiescence [10]. The disease usually resolves rapidly after parturition, often with remaining postinflammatory hyperpigmentation after pustules heal, but usually without residual psoriatic plaques [22, 26]. Scarring is absent unless the lesions are severely excoriated or secondarily infected [22]. The disease may occasionally persist long after delivery [12].

13.5
Laboratory Findings

Leukocytosis with a neutrophil increase and a relative lymphopenia and an elevated sedimentation rate are expected during a severe exacerbation [9, 19, 22]. Other abnormal laboratory findings include hypoalbuminemia, increased levels of blood urea nitrogen, and increased levels of uric acid [19]. Pus from the lesions is sterile, as are blood cultures except when there is a secondary infection [22]. Some cases have shown albuminuria with red and white blood cells in the urine of these patients [9].

Several cases have been found to be associated with hypocalcemia and hyperphosphatemia as a manifestation of hypoparathyroidism [2,26]. In the report by Moslein [17], hypocalcemia or tetany was found in nearly 50% of 113 cases reviewed [14]. Accordingly, there were some investigators that considered hypocalcemia to be essential for the diagnosis of this entity [4,23].

Hypocalcemia may be relative, secondary to decreased levels of albumin [15]. The hypoalbuminemia can stem from the effects of the severe disease itself or be a normal physiologic effect of pregnancy, as a decrease of 1 gm/dL in serum proteins is normal in pregnancy [22]. When IH is associated with hypoparathyroidism, the hypocalcemia is absolute [15]. Measuring the free-ionized calcium is a more reliable method than measuring total calcium, but when this measurement is unavailable, one can use the following formula [22]: Percentage bound $Ca^{2+} = 8[albumin] + 2[globulins] + 3$.

13.6
Histopathology

The picture may be impossible to differentiate from that of pustular psoriasis [22]. The typical lesion is the spongiform pustule of Kogoj, which is a spongiform cavity arising in the epidermis by collapse of keratinocytes, and which becomes filled with polymorphonuclear neutrophils that have migrated from the papillary capillaries to the stratum malpighii of the epidermis [4, 11, 22, 23]. This lesion usually remains a microabscess in psoriasis vulgaris, but in IH it enlarges to huge proportions [22]. This blister is sterile [1]. As it enlarges, loss of the spongiform architecture is evident, and an intraepidermal unilocular macropustule is formed, corresponding to the visible lesion [22].

These lesions are associated with a moderately dense inflammatory infiltrate of lymphocytes, histiocytes, and neutrophils surrounding the superficial dermal blood vessels [4, 23]. Additional findings that may also be seen are similar to those of psoriasis and include parakeratosis, regular elongation of the rete ridges, and migration of mononuclear cells from dermal capillaries into the epidermis [11, 27]. Direct and indirect immunofluorescence tests are negative [27].

13.7
Physiopathology

The cause of IH is still unknown [26]. It may be a distinct entity [15], although because of its clinical resemblance to pustular psoriasis and the extremely low levels of skin-derived anti-leukoproteinase found in patients, most authorities now consider it a variant of acute pustular psoriasis. This variant is said to occur in a latent psoriatic, triggered by a metabolic state, such as hypoparathyroidism or the hormonal environment of pregnancy [14, 16, 22, 27].

The relation to hypoparathyroidism was clearly evident when this condition was observed after accidental removal of the parathyroids during thyroidectomy [14]. Pregnancy leads to increased demand for calcium in the last trimester; thus, it may in itself cause frank hypocalcemia in patients with latent hypoparathyroidism [22]. In turn, hypocalcemia has been shown to exacerbate generalized pustular psoriasis [3]. However, there are reports of plaque-type psoriasis being alleviated during pregnancy (see Section 7.2). Therefore, the physiopathologic relationship between IH and pregnancy is unclear [27].

13.8
Differential Diagnosis

The only other dermatitis of pregnancy having a pustule as a primary lesion is autoimmune progesterone dermatitis [5]. As there are only sparse reported cases of this entity, differentiation should cause little difficulty [27]. In the impetiginized state, IH can resemble herpes gestationis, but biopsy and direct immunofluorescence should differentiate the two disorders [27]. Other diseases that should also be included in the differential diagnosis are erythema multiforme and IgA pemphigus [26].

Clinically, IH bears a close resemblance to pustular conditions such as pustular psoriasis, subcorneal pustular dermatosis, and infectious impetigo [22, 26]. Others think it might be a variant of dermatitis herpetiformis [23]. Clinical differentiation among IH, dermatitis herpetiformis, and pustular psoriasis may on occasion be very difficult or impossible [26]. There are several features typical to IH that may serve as important clues to help differentiate among these diseases. These are summarized in Box 13.1.

13.9
Treatment

The treatment of choice is administration of systemic oral corticosteroids, which has a variable response [1, 23]. They are usually effective at the relatively low dosage of 15–30 mg prednisone per day of, but sometimes dosages up to 60 mg/day are needed to prevent new pustules [18, 22]. This regimen, together with cautious use of systemic antibiotics in super-infected cases, has changed the prognosis of the disease, and nowadays it is not considered to be fatal [22]. Prednisone dosages should be slowly tapered, as rapid removal may

> **Box 13.1** Typical features of impetigo herpetiformis to help in differential diagnosis [22, 26]
>
> ⟩ The primary lesion is a sterile intraepidermal pustule.
> ⟩ Pruritus, if present, is mild.
> ⟩ Severe systemic symptoms are common.
> ⟩ There is no familial or hereditary tendency.
> ⟩ The course of the disease is stormy.
> ⟩ There are unique triggering factors (pregnancy and hypoparathyroidism).
> ⟩ Immunofluorescence tests are negative.

precipitate increased disease activity [18]. Topical corticosteroids have been used beneficially in some cases [13]. Antibiotics may be given also prophylactically, to prevent secondary infections of open lesions [13].

Serum calcium and albumin levels should be followed [18], as well as cultures in order to rule out sepsis and cutaneous infection [18]. Supportive therapy should be employed with fluid and maintenance of electrolyte balance and correction of hypocalcemia if present [6,27].

ACTH has also been used by some authors to avoid possible fetal adrenal suppression [4]. This treatment was successful in controlling skin lesions, but the dose necessary to do so was associated with mineralocorticoid side effects [4]. Sulfapyridine and sulfones have not been helpful in the treatment of this condition [22], in contrast to their beneficial effects in dermatitis herpetiformis and Sneddon–Wilkinson disease [22]. One report of IH associated with hypocalcemia described a dramatic response to parenterally administered 100 mg calcium and 10,000 units of vitamin D daily after treatment with systemic steroids had failed [2]. The eruption may also respond to gonadotropic hormones [14]. In the nonpregnant patient, success with methotrexate and tetracycline has been reported [9]. In severe cases, termination of pregnancy has also been advocated [26].

13.10
Prognosis

The maternal prognosis associated with this disease in von Hebra's time, prior to the use of corticosteroids and antibiotics, was very poor and the mortality rate has been reported to be as high as 70–90% [26]. Patients succumbed within days or weeks secondary to the development of hyperthermia, prostration, renal failure, or heart failure [14, 27]. Fortunately, this dark prognosis is now a thing of the past [22].

In the past, abortion, stillbirth, and neonatal death were frequent [27]. In contrast to maternal prognosis, fetal prognosis may still be poor, as decreased placental function resulting in increased frequency of stillbirths has been reported despite adequate control of the disease with steroids [4, 14]. The more severe and long-standing the IH, the greater are the risks for placental insufficiency [21]. Fetal surveillance is necessary, and delivery is advised by induction of labor or cesarean section as soon as there is evidence of fetal pulmonary maturity when the maternal condition worsens [13, 19].

Summary

> Impetigo herpetiformis is probably a variant of pustular psoriasis of von Zumbusch appearing in pregnancy.
> It is a very rare entity, with fewer than 200 cases reported in the literature.
> It starts with erythematous plaques with pustular margins in intertriginous areas that later coalesce to involve all the body skin, sparing the face, feet, and hands.
> It is accompanied by severe systemic symptoms, with hypocalcemia leading to tetany and delirium.
> Laboratory findings include mainly leukocytosis, hypocalcemia, and hyperphosphatemia.
> Histopathologic features include the typical spongiform pustule of Kogoj, and may show characteristic lesions of psoriasis.
> The main differential diagnoses include dermatitis herpetiformis and pustular eruptions such as pustular psoriasis, subcorneal pustular dermatosis, and infectious impetigo.
> The treatment of choice is orally administered prednisone, 15–30 mg/day.
> Prognosis for the mother is nowadays very good. Placental insufficiency may lead to stillbirths, therefore fetal surveillance is necessary and induction of labor is advocated in severe cases.

References

1. Al-Fares SI, Jones SV, Black MM (2001) The specific dermatoses of pregnancy: a re-appraisal. J Eur Acad Dermatol Venereol 15:197–206
2. Bajaj AK, Swarup V, Gupta OP et al (1977) Impetigo herpetiformis. Dermatologica 155:292–295
3. Baker H, Ryan TJ (1968) Generalized pustular psoriasis. A clinical and epidemiological study of 104 cases. Br J Dermatol 80:771–793
4. Beveridge GW, Harkness RA, Livingstone JR (1966) Impetigo herpetiformis in two successive pregnancies. Br J Dermatol 78:106–112
5. Bierman SM (1973) Autoimmune progesterone dermatitis of pregnancy. Arch Dermatol 107:896–901
6. Callen JP (1984) Pregnancy's effects on the skin. Common and uncommon changes. Postgrad Med 75:138–145
7. Champiom R (1959) Generalized putular psoriasis. Br J Dermatol 71:384
8. Cohen LM (1998) Dermatoses of pregnancy. West J Med 169:223–224
9. Dacus JV (1990) Pruritus in pregnancy. Clin Obstet Gynecol 33:738–745
10. Errickson CV, Matus NR (1994) Skin disorders of pregnancy. Am Fam Physician 49:605–610
11. Eudy SF, Baker GF (1990) Dermatopathology for the obstetrician. Clin Obstet Gynecol 33:728–737
12. Gligora M, Kolacio Z (1982) Hormonal treatment of impetigo herpetiformis. Br J Dermatol 107:253

13. Hayashi RH (1990) Bullous dermatoses and prurigo of pregnancy. Clin Obstet Gynecol 33:746–753
14. Hellreich P (1974) The skin changes of pregnancy. Cutis 13:82–86
15. Katzenellenbogen I, Feuerman E (1966) Psoriasis pustulosa and impetigo hepetiformis in two successive pregnancies. Acta Derm Venereol 46:86
16. McKenzie AW (1971) Skin disorders in pregnancy. Practitioner 206:773–780
17. Moslein P (1959) Impetigo herpetiformis, psoriasis pustulosa, acrodermatitis continua Hallopeau. Arch Klin Exp Dermatol 208:410–458
18. Murray JC (1990) Pregnancy and the skin. Dermatol Clin 8:327–334
19. Oosterling RJ, Nobrega RE, Du Boeuff JA et al (1978) Impetigo herpetiformis or generalized pustular psoriasis? Arch Dermatol 114:1527–1529
20. Ott F, Krakowski A, Tur E et al (1982) Impetigo herpetiformis with lowered serum level of vitamin D and its diminished intestinal absorption. Dermatologica 164:360–365
21. Oumeish OY, Farraj SE, Bataineh AS (1982) Some aspects of impetigo herpetiformis. Arch Dermatol 118:103–105
22. Sasseville D, Wilkinson RD, Schnader JY (1981) Dermatoses of pregnancy. Int J Dermatol 20:223–241
23. Sauer GC, Geha BJ (1961) Impetigo herpetiformis. Report of a case treated with corticosteroid-review of the literature. Arch Dermatol 83:119–126
24. Sodhi VK, Sausker WF (1988) Dermatoses of pregnancy. Am Fam Physician 37:131–138
25. Tunzi M, Gray GR (2007) Common skin conditions during pregnancy. Am Fam Physician 75:211–218
26. Wade TR, Wade SL, Jones HE (1978) Skin changes and diseases associated with pregnancy. Obstet Gynecol 52:233–242
27. Winton GB, Lewis CW (1982) Dermatoses of pregnancy. J Am Acad Dermatol 6:977–998

Autoimmune Progesterone Dermatitis of Pregnancy

14

14.1
Definition

Autoimmune progesterone dermatitis of pregnancy was described only once in the medical literature, and relates to a nonpruritic, acneiform eruption triggered by pregnancy due to hypersensitivity to endogenous progesterone. This entity recurs in succeeding pregnancies and is connected to spontaneous abortions [8].

14.2
Introduction

In 1973 a single patient was described by Bierman [1], who in two consecutive pregnancies developed an odd acneiform eruption of the limbs and buttocks associated with polyarthritis. The patient had a positive intradermal skin test to progesterone [10]. Both pregnancies resulted in spontaneous abortions. Bierman [1] named the disease "autoimmune progesterone dermatitis of pregnancy."

The more common autoimmune progesterone dermatitis, which is not related to pregnancy, has been known for many years [10, 11]. This disease is characterized by a pruritic, vesiculobullous or urticarial eruption, which develops on the trunk or extremities in a repeated pattern 7–10 days before each menstruation period [7, 9]. In many cases the triggering factor is the use of progesterone-containing oral medications which may sensitize the body to endogenous progesterone [10]. Intradermal skin testing with progesterone may be positive, and the disease can be controlled with estrogen therapy [7] or by oophorectomy [9].

Bierman's case is the first and, fortunately, the only one reported in which lesions appeared in pregnancy [1], and it seems to be a distinct clinical entity [10].

A. Ingber, *Obstetric Dermatology,*
DOI: 10.1007/978-3-540-88399-9, © Springer-Verlag Berlin Heidelberg 2009

14.3
Clinical Presentation

In Bierman's patient, a 25-year-old East Indian woman, an explosive acneiform eruption occurred in the first 2 weeks of pregnancy in two consecutive pregnancies [1]. The dermatitis first appeared as nonpruritic follicular and perifollicular comedones, papules, and pustules [1]. The papules were 0.5–2 mm in diameter, firm, and tender, and formed groups [1]. There was no vesiculation or excoriation [1]. Later in the course of the disease, larger, firm, turbid and tender pustules on an inflammatory base appeared [1]. As the papules matured, they developed a psoriasiform scale [1]. An area of postinflammatory hyperpigmentation was left after involution of the lesions [1]. Lesions occurred in sites not usually seen with acne, first acrally on the fingers, arms, and legs, and rapidly spreading to involve the buttocks. Interestingly, they were associated with polyarthritis involving the metacarpophalangeal joints, wrists, knees, and ankles [1].

A coincidental intestinal colonization with *Giardia lamblia* was detected during the second pregnancy. It was treated without any effect on the skin disease [1].

The condition reappeared in two succeeding pregnancies, both of which terminated in spontaneous abortions followed by gradual slow resolution of the skin lesions [1]. No premenstrual flares occurred; however, during a disease-free interval, the patient was challenged with an oral contraceptive and the dermatitis and arthritis recurred [1].

14.4
Laboratory Findings

A laboratory workup revealed elevated serum levels of IgG and IgM [1]. An unusually high eosinophilia of 53% was found, presumably due to the coexisting intestinal giardiasis. It later went down to 14% after eradication of this parasite, and then seemed to correspond to the clinical course of the disease [1].

Cultures grew *Proteus*, *Klebsiella*, and enterobacteria species when taken from the skin, whereas they grew *Escherichia coli* and *Staphylococcus aureus* when taken from a skin pustule [1].

Intradermal skin tests were performed with both estrogen and progesterone [1]. At 48 h, the patient *developed* a large painful abscess at the site of progesterone injection [1]. Estrogen injection did not elicit any response [1]. Direct and indirect immunofluorescence tests were negative, and no serum antibody was found [1].

14.5
Histopathology

Biopsy of a clinical lesion revealed an acanthotic epidermis with focal spongiosis, and exocytosis of a chronic inflammatory infiltrate including lymphocytes and histiocytes [1]. A moderately dense infiltrate composed mainly of eosinophils was present at all levels of the dermis in both a perivascular and an interstitial distribution [1]. In the subcutaneous tissue, a pattern of lobular panniculitis was present with a large number of eosinophils, lymphocytes, and histiocytes, and with abscess formation [1]. Some specimens also revealed intraepidermal abscess formation composed almost entirely of eosinophils [1].

14.6
Physiopathology

As stated previously, many cases have been reported of vesicular [9], urticarial [4], or eczematous [5] dermatitis worsened in the premenstrual period and associated with a positive delayed skin test to progesterone [8].

This case, the first to be described in pregnancy, follows the same biological and clinical pattern of autoimmune progesterone dermatitis [8]. Owing to the reduplication of the skin lesion postpartum by oral contraceptives, the positive reaction to treatment with aqueous conjugated estrogens, and the reproduction of the histopathologic findings at the site of intradermal progesterone injection, it is reasonable to assume that it is caused by a hypersensitivity reaction to endogenous progesterone [3, 8]. However, it is not clear how this sensitization occurred or what biochemical mechanisms are involved [10]. Both premenopausal and postmenopausal women have been reported to have similar eruptions [2]. Although affected women usually have a history of previous exogenous progesterone exposure, cases of endogenous progesterone hypersensitivity have been reported [6].

Bierman's patient never had premenstrual exacerbations of her dermatitis, although she had flares after skin testing with progesterone and on a low-dose oral contraceptive (norinyl) whose hormonal levels are comparable to those seen at the time of ovulation [8]. A study of the patient's lymphocytes for mitogenic response to her progesterone was negative [1]. It should be noted that there are patients with progesterone-induced dermatitis who improve with the high progesterone levels during pregnancy [8]. In conclusion, the precise dynamics of progesterone dermatitis is still far from clear [8].

14.7
Differential Diagnosis

Acne fulminans, halogenoderma, or acneiform drug eruptions can produce a similar skin eruption, and may have to be ruled out [8]. The uncommonness of autoimmune progesterone dermatitis makes it unknown to most practitioners; therefore, it might be confused with any of the other dermatoses of pregnancy [8], although its clinical presentation, biological background, and histopathologic characteristics are typical enough to permit accurate diagnosis [8].

14.8
Treatment

The patient's condition was investigated and treated only in the postabortum period [1]. Ovulation was blocked with 1.25 mg of conjugated equine estrogen given for 21 days a month with rapid improvement of the dermatitis [1]. Such treatment is probably ineffective in pregnancy. Thus, an adequate treatment for the prepartum stage of the disease is still wanting [8].

14.9
Prognosis

As mentioned earlier, in the single case report described this condition had a 100% fetal mortality, as both pregnancies terminated in spontaneous abortions [1]. It is still unknown whether these deaths were coincidental or represent fetal ill effects from a severe systemic maternal disease [8].

References

1. Bierman SM (1973) Autoimmune progesterone dermatitis of pregnancy. Arch Dermatol 107:896–901
2. Bolaji II, O'Dwyer EM (1992) Post-menopausal cyclic eruptions: autoimmune progesterone dermatitis. Eur J Obstet Gynecol Reprod Biol 47:169–171
3. Dahdah MJ, Kibbi AG (2006) Less well-defined dermatoses of pregnancy. Clin Dermatol 24:118–121
4. Farah FS, Shbaklu Z (1971) Autoimmune progesterone urticaria. J Allergy Clin Immunol 48:257–261
5. Jones WN, Gordon VH (1969) Auto-immune progesterone eczema. An endogenous progesterone hypersensitivity. Arch Dermatol 99:57–59
6. Moody BR, Schatten S (1997) Autoimmune progesterone dermatitis: onset in a women without previous exogenous progesterone exposure. South Med J 90:845–846
7. Nouri K, Bowes L, Chartier T et al (1999) Combination treatment of melasma with pulsed CO2 laser followed by Q-switched alexandrite laser: a pilot study. Dermatol Surg 25:494–497
8. Sasseville D, Wilkinson RD, Schnader JY (1981) Dermatoses of pregnancy. Int J Dermatol 20:223–241
9. Shelley WB, Cohen W (1964) Stria migrans. Arch Dermatol 90:193–194
10. Winton GB, Lewis CW (1982) Dermatoses of pregnancy. J Am Acad Dermatol 6:977–998
11. Zondek B, Bromberg V (1945) Endocrine allergy. I. Allergic sensitivity to endogenous hormones. J Allergy 16:1

Linear IgM Dermatosis of Pregnancy

Linear IgM dermatosis of pregnancy (LMDP) was described by Alcalay et al. [1] in a single case report in a 39-year-old woman. It was characterized by intensely pruritic, red, follicular papules and pustules on the abdomen, forearms, thighs and legs (Figs. 15.1, 15.2). The rash did not respond to topically applied calamine lotion and oral antihistamines [1]. The histologic features were compatible with folliculitis [1]. A biopsy for direct immunofluorescence revealed bright, dense, linear IgM deposits at the basement membrane zone (BMZ) [1] (Fig. 15.3). Indirect immunofluorescence testing was negative [1]. Lesions began during the 37th week of gestation and resolved within 6 weeks of delivery, and repeat direct immunofluorescence testing after resolution of the rash was negative [1]. The rash did not affect the outcome of the pregnancy [1]. Recently, Pavlovsky Lev, Segal Rina, Michael David (personal communication) from the Department of Dermatology, Rabin Medical Center, Petach–Tiqva, Israel, described a similar case. A 31-year-old woman, in her 30th week of pregnancy, developed a pruritic eruption located on her abdomen, breast, and limbs 1 week following beginning nifedipine therapy for premature contractions (Fig. 15.4). Direct immunofluorescence testing revealed linear IgM deposits at the BMZ (Fig. 15.5). Therapy with nifedipine was discontinued and 3 days later, when notable improvement was seen, she decided to rechallenge herself with nifedipine. The eruption exacerbated in a short time (Fig. 15.6). They concluded that LMDP may be drug-related.

Circulating IgM anti-BMZ antibodies were found on indirect immunofluorescence testing in 10, 12, and 14% of healthy pregnant women, pregnant women with polymorphic eruption of pregnancy and nonpregnant women, respectively [2]. The incidence of IgM deposits at the BMZ in men and nonpregnant women showed no clinical association [3]. They were seen in urticaria, leukocytoclastic vasculitis, pigmented purpuric dermatosis, hypersensitivity dermatitis, folliculitis, paraneoplastic pemphigus, and Grover disease [4]. Therefore, the meaning of the IgM antibodies is unknown, and the existence of LMDP as an entity is debated [3]. Some authors categorize it as a variant of polymorphic eruption of pregnancy or prurigo of pregnancy [5].

A. Ingber, *Obstetric Dermatology*,
DOI: 10.1007/978-3-540-88399-9, © Springer-Verlag Berlin Heidelberg 2009

Fig. 15.1 Linear IgM dermatosis of pregnancy. Many pustules and erythemic papules on the abdomen. Note linea nigra under the umbilicus

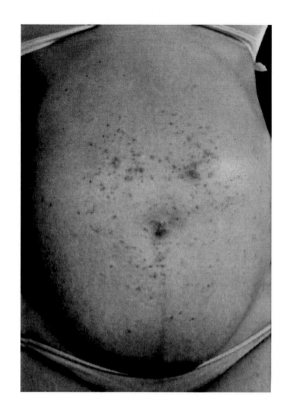

Fig. 15.2 Linear IgM dermatosis of pregnancy. Close view. Pustular rash

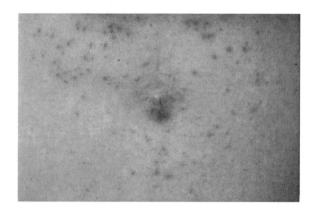

Fig. 15.3 Linear IgM dermatosis of pregnancy. Direct immunofluorescence. Linear IgM along the dermoepidermal junction

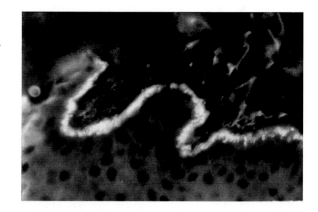

Fig. 15.4 Linear IgM dermatosis of pregnancy. Pustules and vesicles on the abdomen. (Courtesy of Lev Pavlovsky)

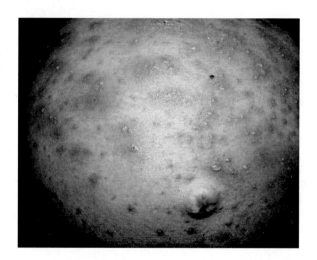

Fig. 15.5 Linear IgM dermatosis of pregnancy. Direct immunofluorescence. Linear deposition of IgM along the dermoepidermal junction. (Courtesy of Lev Pavlovsky)

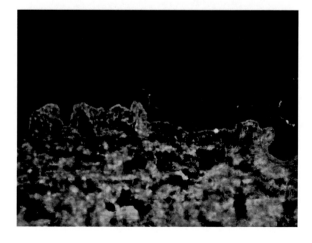

Fig. 15.6 Linear IgM dermatosis of pregnancy. Following rechallenge with nifedipine, there are numerous pustules on the abdomen. (Courtesy of Lev Pavlovsky)

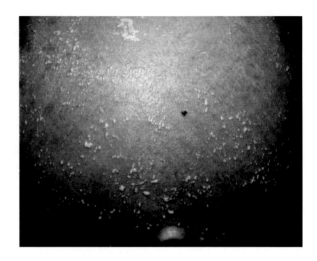

References

1. Alcalay J, Ingber A, Hazaz B et al (1988) Linear IgM dermatosis of pregnancy. J Am Acad Dermatol 18:412–415
2. Borradori L, Didierjean L, Bernard P et al (1995) IgM autoantibodies to 180- and 230- to 240-kd human epidermal proteins in pregnancy. Arch Dermatol 131:43–47
3. Dahdah MJ, Kibbi AG (2006) Less well-defined dermatoses of pregnancy. Clin Dermatol 24:118–121
4. Helm TN, Valenzuela R (1992) Continuous dermoepidermal junction IgM detected by direct immunofluorescence: a report of nine cases. J Am Acad Dermatol 26:203–206
5. Kroumpouzos G, Cohen LM (2001) Dermatoses of pregnancy. J Am Acad Dermatol 45:1–19; quiz 19–22

Prurigo of Pregnancy

16

16.1
Definition

Prurigo of pregnancy (PP) is a relatively common benign skin disease characterized by pruritic papules primarily on the extensor aspects of the extremities. Prognosis for mother and fetus is excellent.

16.2
Introduction

The term "prurigo gestationis" was first introduced by Besnier et al. [4] in 1904 to include all patients with a pregnancy rash, other than herpes gestationis [1]. Later, Nurse [16], in 1968, divided PP into two main groups: "early onset" and "late onset" PP; the latter group apparently included cases of pruritic urticarial papules and plaques of pregnancy (PUPPP) [1].

Nowadays, "prurigo of pregnancy" is a term that encompasses Besnier's prurigo gestationis, Nurse's early-onset form of prurigo, and Spangler's papular dermatosis of pregnancy [19]. PP may be a distinct entity, may represent an unusual variant of PUPPP [8], or may be a simplified labeling of a heterogeneous group, classified together because of broad clinical overlap, incomplete evaluation, and the fact that the pathogenesis has not been identified in any of them [14, 19]. It has been debated whether "linear IgM dermatosis of pregnancy" described by Alcalay et al. [2] should be classified as a distinct entity or whether it may be a variant of PUPPP or PP [18, 19, 23]. In 2006, Ambros-Rudolph et al. [3] proposed reclassifying PP as part of a newly defined disease complex, named "atopic eruption of pregnancy."

A. Ingber, *Obstetric Dermatology*,
DOI: 10.1007/978-3-540-88399-9, © Springer-Verlag Berlin Heidelberg 2009

16.3
Incidence

PP is a relatively common skin disorder during pregnancy [11]. Its incidence varies between one in 300 pregnancies and one in 450 pregnancies [16, 17], and it may account for up to 6% of pregnancy-associated dermatoses [22]. It is probably more common in women with atopic dermatitis, where the severe pruritus results in the development of prurigo lesions [1].

16.4
Clinical Presentation

PP has been reported in all trimesters of pregnancies, but it typically presents during the second or the third trimester, most commonly in the 25th to the 30th week of pregnancy [8, 14, 19].

PP is characterized by small groups of discrete, erythematous or skin-colored papules and nodules, which are extremely itchy, resulting in excoriated lesions. They develop primarily on the extensor surfaces of the arms and legs and on the dorsal aspects of the hands and feet, and occasionally on the abdomen (Figs. 16.1–16.4) [1, 6, 8, 11, 14]. In some cases the lesions may spread to the chest and back [5].

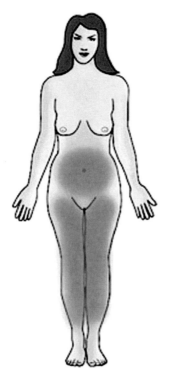

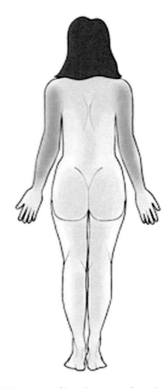

Fig. 16.1 Areas of involvement of prurigo of pregnancy, anterior view

Fig. 16.2 Areas of involvement of prurigo of pregnancy, posterior view

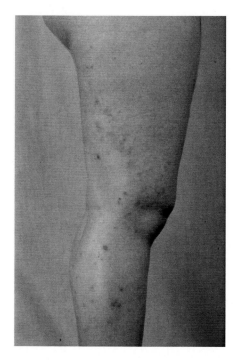

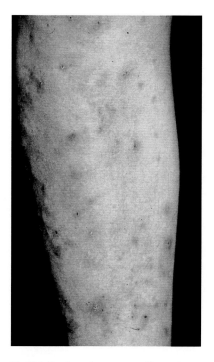

Fig. 16.3 Prurigo of pregnancy. Typical lesions on the lower extremities

Fig. 16.4 Prurigo of pregnancy. Close view. Minute lesions on erythemic papules

The lesions are typically small, 0.5–1 cm in size, with or without a central crust, and the skin surrounding these papules remains normal [1, 19]. The lesions may occasionally appear crusted or eczematous [14, 15]. Pustules may be evident, but vesicles are never seen [14]. The lesions are similar to the ones seen in prurigo nodularis of nonpregnant women [19, 21]. According to the author's personal experience, the nodules in PP are smaller than those in prurigo nodularis and they are not so dark even in patients with dark-colored skin.

The disease runs a protracted course through gestation, and although it commonly resolves after delivery, it may last up to 3 months postpartum [13–15]. Recurrence during subsequent gestations is variable [12, 14, 16, 19].

16.5
Laboratory Findings

Laboratory studies have revealed no abnormalities [5]. Serologic test results are normal [13]. The hormonal aberrations (elevated β-human chorionic gonadotropin and decreased cortisol and estrogen levels) and the gloomy fetal outcome reported by Spangler et al. [20] have not been confirmed by any other studies [15].

16.6
Histopathology

The diagnosis of PP is mainly a clinical one; as a result, a skin biopsy is not always executed [1]. When a biopsy is done, it may show acanthosis with overlying parakeratosis, evidence of excoriation (crusting and fibrin deposition), and a chronic perivascular inflammatory cell infiltrate including lymphocytes, histiocytes, neutrophils, and eosinophils in the upper dermis [13, 14]. Direct and indirect immunofluorescence tests are classically negative [19].

16.7
Physiopathology

The cause of PP is not well understood [11, 19]. Because it is likely that this group is heterogeneous, numerous pathways may be related [19]. The ensuing scratching in response to the pruritus is thought to play a role, although the cause of the pruritus is unknown [10].

PP may be associated with a family history of intrahepatic cholestasis of pregnancy (ICP), and its differentiation from ICP can be challenging [15, 17]. Occasionally, the only differentiating characteristic between the two entities is the absence of primary lesions in ICP [15]. Some authors have suggested that PP and ICP may be different levels of severity of the same disease [7].

PP can resemble atopic dermatitis [11], and Black [5, 13] has suggested that the findings may be the result of ICP in women with an atopic diathesis. This is supported by the fact that many patients with PP have a positive history of atopy (eczema, asthma, and hay fever) and by the elevated level of serum IgE, which is an indicator of atopy, detected in PP patients in two studies [18, 22]. The association with atopy was not confirmed by other studies [17].

16.8
Diagnosis

The primary differential is between a specific dermatosis of pregnancy and the wide varieties of pruritic entities not related to gestation [19]. Bites, arthropods, and especially scabies should be excluded [14, 19]. All patients should undergo studies for normal liver function and serum bile acids [19]. Drug-induced disease should be excluded [19].

16.9
Treatment

PP is annoying, but benign, and treatment is symptomatic [8, 19]. The lesions respond well to moderately to highly potent topical corticosteroids [1, 5, 9]. Other antipruritic agents including oral antihistamines such as chlorpheniramine may be beneficial [1, 11]. The use of translucent polythene adhesive film impregnated with flurandrenolone (Cordran tape) can be supportive to treat a small number of localized discrete lesions [1]. At the Department of Dermatology at Hadassah University Hospital (Jerusalem, Israel), we treated many PP patients with narrowband UVB, 20–30 treatments, with great success (unpublished data).

16.10
Prognosis

PP is a benign disorder with no associated effect on the pregnancy or the newborn baby [1]. The birth weight is normal [22], and the condition usually abates postpartum [14]. Because there is no associated fetal morbidity or mortality, there is no indication for intervention [8, 19].

Summary

> Prurigo of pregnancy encompasses Besnier's prurigo gestationis, Nurse's early-onset form of prurigo, and Spangler's papular dermatosis of pregnancy.
> The incidence is approximately one in 300 pregnancies.
> It presents as pruritic papules primarily on the extensor aspects of the extremities.
> The cause is unknown, but may be related to the effect of scratching on the skin of atopic women.
> Treatment is symptomatic with topical corticosteroids, oral antihistamines, or narrowband UVB.
> There is normal maternal and fetal prognosis.

References

1. Al-Fares SI, Jones SV, Black MM (2001) The specific dermatoses of pregnancy: a re-appraisal. J Eur Acad Dermatol Venereol 15:197–206
2. Alcalay J, Ingber A, Hazaz B et al (1988) Linear IgM dermatosis of pregnancy. J Am Acad Dermatol 18:412–415
3. Ambros-Rudolph CM, Mullegger RR, Vaughan-Jones SA et al (2006) The specific dermatoses of pregnancy revisited and reclassified: results of a retrospective two-center study on 505 pregnant patients. J Am Acad Dermatol 54:395–404
4. Besnier E, Brocq L, Jacquet L (1904) La pratique dermatologique. Masson et Cie, Paris
5. Black MM (1989) Prurigo of pregnancy, papular dermatitis of pregnancy, and pruritic folliculitis of pregnancy. Semin Dermatol 8:23–25
6. Black MM (1997) Progress and new directions in the investigation of the specific dermatoses of pregnancy. Keio J Med 46:40–41

7. Bos JD (1999) Reappraisal of dermatoses of pregnancy. Lancet 354:1140
8. Cohen LM (1998) Dermatoses of pregnancy. West J Med 169:223–224
9. Dahdah MJ, Kibbi AG (2006) Less well-defined dermatoses of pregnancy. Clin Dermatol 24:118–121
10. Errickson CV, Matus NR (1994) Skin disorders of pregnancy. Am Fam Physician 49:605–610
11. Fuhrman L (2000) Common dermatoses of pregnancy. J Perinat Neonatal Nurs 14:1–16
12. Hayashi RH (1990) Bullous dermatoses and prurigo of pregnancy. Clin Obstet Gynecol 33:746–753
13. Holmes RC, Black MM (1983) The specific dermatoses of pregnancy. J Am Acad Dermatol 8:405–412
14. Kroumpouzos G, Cohen LM (2001) Dermatoses of pregnancy. J Am Acad Dermatol 45:1–19; quiz 19–22
15. Kroumpouzos G, Cohen LM (2003) Specific dermatoses of pregnancy: an evidence-based systematic review. Am J Obstet Gynecol 188:1083–1092
16. Nurse DS (1968) Prurigo of pregnancy. Australas J Dermatol 9:258–267
17. Roger D, Vaillant L, Fignon A et al (1994) Specific pruritic diseases of pregnancy. A prospective study of 3192 pregnant women. Arch Dermatol 130:734–739
18. Sasseville D, Wilkinson RD, Schnader JY (1981) Dermatoses of pregnancy. Int J Dermatol 20:223–241
19. Shornick JK (1998) Dermatoses of pregnancy. Semin Cutan Med Surg 17:172–181
20. Spangler AS, Reddy W, Bardawil WA et al (1962) Papular dermatitis of pregnancy. A new clinical entity? JAMA 181:577–581
21. Vaughan Jones SA, Black MM (1999) Pregnancy dermatoses. J Am Acad Dermatol 40:233–241
22. Vaughan Jones SA, Hern S, Nelson-Piercy C et al (1999) A prospective study of 200 women with dermatoses of pregnancy correlating clinical findings with hormonal and immunopathological profiles. Br J Dermatol 141:71–81
23. Velthuis PJ, de Jong MC, Kruis MH (1988) Is there a linear IgM dermatosis? Significance of linear IgM junctional staining in cutaneous immunopathology. Acta Derm Venereol 68:8–14

Pruritic Folliculitis of Pregnancy

17

17.1
Definition

Pruritic folliculitis of pregnancy (PFP) is a benign, self-limiting condition, characterized by pruritic follicular papules involving mainly the upper back and abdomen and extremities.

17.2
Introduction

PFP was initially described in 1981 by Zoberman and Farmer [22]. They reported six pregnant women who presented with sterile pruritic papular folliculitis in the fourth to ninth months of pregnancy that resolved spontaneously at or after delivery. Since the original description, many cases have been reported [4, 9–12, 16, 20, 21].

Although it is apparently not dangerous to both the mother and the fetus, it might be a variant of pruritic urticarial papules and plaques of pregnancy (PUPPP), with evidence of folliculitis on histologic examination [6], or a form of acne/folliculitis that occurs in pregnancy due to hormonal changes [7].

17.3
Incidence

The condition seems to be more common than previously thought, as it is likely that there is a lack of awareness among dermatologists, and many cases of PFP are undiagnosed or misdiagnosed as acne, microbial folliculitis, or PUPPP [13, 14]. It seems to be as common as herpes gestationis and prurigo of pregnancy in the UK, with an estimated incidence of

A. Ingber, *Obstetric Dermatology*,
DOI: 10.1007/978-3-540-88399-9, © Springer-Verlag Berlin Heidelberg 2009

17

one in 3,000 pregnancies [17]. In a series of 200 women with skin rashes during pregnancy, 14 of them (7%) had PFP [20].

17.4
Clinical Presentation

This disorder begins in the fourth to ninth months of pregnancy [22]. Masses of mono-morphous 3–5-mm follicular erythematous papules with sterile pustules characterize PFP [7, 8, 22]. The lesions are easily excoriated [8], and are centered on hair follicles [1]. The lesions appear in a generalized distribution in most patients, involving mainly the upper abdomen and back, but can also spread to the legs and arms (Figs. 17.1, 17.2) [1, 3, 22]. The clinical appearance of this eruption strongly resembles the monomorphic type of steroid-induced acne [11, 22]. Contrary to its name, pruritus is not a major feature [18].

Generally, the eruption runs a benign course, and resolves either shortly after delivery or within 1 month of delivery [1, 7, 22]. It does not tend to recur in subsequent pregnancies [1].

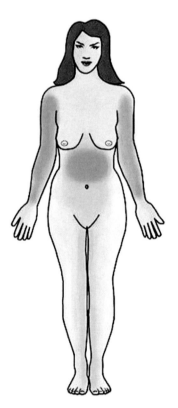
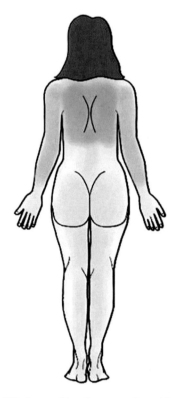

Fig. 17.1 Areas of involvement of pruritic fol-liculitis of pregnancy, anterior view

Fig. 17.2 Areas of involvement of pruritic fol-liculitis of pregnancy, posterior view

17.5
Histopathology

In a small number of cases histopathologic examination was reported to be diagnostic of acute folliculitis, with perifollicular neutrophilic infiltrate. In most cases, the changes are nonspecific and consist of excoriations and a perivascular lymphohistiocytic inflammatory infiltrate [1]. Staining for organisms is invariably negative; however, rarely, Gram-positive cocci or bacilli have been reported [1, 11, 20, 22].

Direct immunofluorescence tests for deposition of immunoglobulins and complement are negative [11, 12, 22].

17.6
Physiopathology

Although the exact cause of PFP is unclear, it has been hypothesized to be hormonal since the lesions disappear within 1 month following delivery [8]. Some have described this eruption as hormonally-induced acne, caused by end-organ hypersensitivity to increased serum levels of sex hormones arising during pregnancy, based on the similarity in the clinical appearance between PFP and monomorphic type of acne occurring after the administration of systemic corticosteroids or progestogens [2, 11, 15, 21]. There has been little additional evidence in favor of this hypothesis [3, 16].

Wilkinson et al. [21] reported one case of PFP in which levels of serum androgens were elevated. However, a later report of 12 cases of PFP showed no significant increase in levels of serum androgens (testosterone, dehydroepiandrosterone sulfate, androstenedione, and sex hormone binding globulin) when compared with those of normal pregnant controls [19]. One report showed an outcome with a male-to-female ratio of 2:1, but the meaning of this remains uncertain [1, 20].

There is no evidence of any immunologic abnormalities in this condition [20]. Association with intrahepatic cholestasis has been reported in one case [9], but this association has not been confirmed by other reports [14].

Some authors have suggested that PFP should be included within the spectrum of "polymorphic eruption of pregnancy" [3]. Follicular lesions have been reported in PUPPP [5], and distinction between the two entities can be difficult [14].

17.7
Diagnosis

The differential diagnosis of PFP includes an infectious folliculitis, which can be excluded by cultures and special stains [13]. Other differentials may include one of the specific dermatoses of pregnancy such as PUPPP, herpes gestationis, and prurigo of pregnancy [13].

17.8
Treatment

The treatment of PFP is supportive, as the eruption is mostly asymptomatic and usually resolves after delivery [8, 13]; mid-potency topical corticosteroids and oral antihistamines have been used with little benefit in most patients [7, 8]. Treatment with topical creams containing a mixture of 10% benzoyl peroxide and 1% hydrocortisone has been reported to be beneficial [3, 22]. Topical antifungals as well as topical and systemic antibiotics have not proven to be successful [12]. One case of successful treatment of PFP with narrow-band UVB phototherapy after 20 treatments has been reported [16].

17.9
Prognosis

PFP is a self-limiting disorder, and no increased maternal or fetal morbidity was described [22]. However, one prospective study of 14 patients showed a predominance of male babies (2:1) and a statistically significant reduced fetal birth weight in women with PFP [20]. PFP has been associated with premature delivery in one case [16].

Summary

› Pruritic folliculitis of pregnancy was described for the first time in 1981 by Zoberman and Farmer.
› It has an estimated incidence of one in 3,000 pregnancies, but the condition is probably underestimated.
› It is characterized by pruritic follicular papules involving mainly the upper back and abdomen and extremities, presenting during the second and third trimesters.
› It may be a form of acne/folliculitis appearing in pregnancy owing to hormonal modifications.
› Treatment is supportive, and may include a mixture of benzoyl peroxide and hydrocortisone.
› Maternal and fetal outcomes are probably normal.

References

1. Al-Fares SI, Jones SV, Black MM (2001) The specific dermatoses of pregnancy: a re-appraisal. J Eur Acad Dermatol Venereol 15:197–206
2. Black M, Stephens C (1989) The specific dermatoses of pregnancy: the British perspective. Adv Dermatol 7:105–127

3. Black MM (1989) Prurigo of pregnancy, papular dermatitis of pregnancy, and pruritic folliculitis of pregnancy. Semin Dermatol 8:23–25
4. Borradori L, Saurat JH (1994) Specific dermatoses of pregnancy. Toward a comprehensive view? Arch Dermatol 130:778–780
5. Borrego L (2000) Follicular lesions in polymorphic eruption of pregnancy. J Am Acad Dermatol 42:146
6. Callen JP (1984) Pregnancy's effects on the skin. Common and uncommon changes. Postgrad Med 75:138–145
7. Cohen LM (1998) Dermatoses of pregnancy. West J Med 169:223–224
8. Dacus JV (1990) Pruritus in pregnancy. Clin Obstet Gynecol 33:738–745
9. Esteve E, Vaillant L, Bacq Y et al (1992) Pruritic folliculitis of pregnancy: role of associated intrahepatic cholestasis? Ann Dermatol Venereol 119:37–40
10. Fox GN (1989) Pruritic folliculitis of pregnancy. Am Fam Physician 39:189–193
11. Holmes RC, Black MM (1983) The specific dermatoses of pregnancy. J Am Acad Dermatol 8:405–412
12. Kroumpouzos G, Cohen LM (2000) Pruritic folliculitis of pregnancy. J Am Acad Dermatol 43:132–134
13. Kroumpouzos G, Cohen LM (2001) Dermatoses of pregnancy. J Am Acad Dermatol 45:1–19; quiz 19–22
14. Kroumpouzos G, Cohen LM (2003) Specific dermatoses of pregnancy: an evidence-based systematic review. Am J Obstet Gynecol 188:1083–1092
15. Murray JC (1990) Pregnancy and the skin. Dermatol Clin 8:327–334
16. Reed J, George S (1999) Pruritic folliculitis of pregnancy treated with narrowband (TL-01) ultraviolet B phototherapy. Br J Dermatol 141:177–179
17. Roger D, Vaillant L, Fignon A et al (1994) Specific pruritic diseases of pregnancy. A prospective study of 3192 pregnant women. Arch Dermatol 130:734–739
18. Tunzi M, Gray GR (2007) Common skin conditions during pregnancy. Am Fam Physician 75:211–218
19. Vaughan Jones SA, Hern S, Black MM (1999) Neutrophil folliculitis and serum androgen levels. Clin Exp Dermatol 24:392–395
20. Vaughan Jones SA, Hern S, Nelson-Piercy C et al (1999) A prospective study of 200 women with dermatoses of pregnancy correlating clinical findings with hormonal and immunopathological profiles. Br J Dermatol 141:71–81
21. Wilkinson SM, Buckler H, Wilkinson N et al (1995) Androgen levels in pruritic folliculitis of pregnancy. Clin Exp Dermatol 20:234–236
22. Zoberman E, Farmer ER (1981) Pruritic folliculitis of pregnancy. Arch Dermatol 117:20–22

Pruritic Urticarial Papules and Plaques of Pregnancy

18

18.1
Definition

Pruritic urticarial papules and plaques of pregnancy (PUPPP) is a benign, extremely pruritic, inflammatory eruption of the third trimester of primigravida pregnancies, characterized by urticarial papules and plaques localized first to the abdomen [2, 27, 53]. It clears at delivery and it is the most common of the gestational dermatoses [53].

18.2
Introduction

This benign eruption of late pregnancy was first reported by Lawley et al. [42] in April 1979, and they descriptively coined the term "pruritic urticarial papules and plaques of pregnancy." They performed a thorough investigation of seven cases, but they probably did not describe a new entity. This entity was initially reported by Bourne [13] as toxemic rash of pregnancy in 1962. The terminology used by Bourne is probably a misnomer, as it was not associated with preeclampsia, and therefore the term has been little used [2]. Nurse's late-onset prurigo gestationis described in 1968 [46] also closely corresponds to PUPPP [53].

The new term has benefited from modern investigative procedures and PUPPP has quickly become a widely recognized entity, and shortly after the article by Lawley et al. had been published several other authors reported similar cases [1, 16, 60, 63]. They found the descriptive title to be more useful from a clinical standpoint and not to be misleading [63].

In 1982 the British investigators Holmes and Black suggested that the term "polymorphic eruption of pregnancy" (PEP) be used to cover the whole spectrum of clinical presentations that include urticarial wheals, papules, erythematous plaques, vesicles, and target lesions [32]. This entity was meant to unite together PUPPP, Bourne's toxemic rash of pregnancy, Besnier's prurigo, and Nurse's late-onset prurigo gestationis [33]. This

A. Ingber, *Obstetric Dermatology*,
DOI: 10.1007/978-3-540-88399-9, © Springer-Verlag Berlin Heidelberg 2009

18

terminology is favored throughout Europe, but has not gained universal support [2, 56], and the term "pruritic urticarial papules and plaques of pregnancy" is still in use especially in the USA [2]. PUPPP and PEP represent identical dermatoses [2].

18.3
Incidence

PUPPP has a worldwide distribution [2]. The disease has a benign nature, and this may lead to difficulty in assessing the exact incidence, as it is probably grossly underreported or overlooked; however, it is by far the most common of the gestational dermatoses [2, 15, 29, 42]. PUPPP has been estimated to occur in one out of 120–300 pregnancies [10, 13, 21, 52].

18.4
Clinical Presentation

The skin eruption usually begins in the third trimester, characteristically between 36 and 39 weeks of the first pregnancy [21, 43, 63]. The average time of onset is the 36th week of gestation [43]. Rarely it may occur as early as the first trimester or as late as the immediate postpartum period (usually within the first 2 weeks after delivery) [21].

Erythematous, pruritic papules that coalesce into erythematous urticarial plaques typically develop suddenly symmetrically on the abdomen [1, 26, 42, 56] (Figs. 18.1, 18.2) Typical individual papules are 1–2 mm in diameter, may be encircled by a narrow pale halo, and blanch without difficulty on application of pressure [21]. In 20% of cases, target lesions that can look almost like those of erythema multiforme may appear [21]. Annular or polycyclic erythematous areas are seen in 18% of cases [32, 41, 46]. These lesions may be clinically indistinguishable from those seen in the very early stages of herpes gestationis (HG) [15, 24, 32, 42, 46, 57]. Purpura is occasionally seen [39].

The most prominent characteristic is the distribution of the lesions [32, 41, 46]. Initially, they are confined to the lower abdominal striae in two thirds of cases, sparing the periumbilical area (in contrast to HG) (Figs. 18.3, 18.4), but the eruption may spread peripherally over a few days to involve a large cutaneous surface, including the thighs, buttocks, flanks, breasts, back, lower thorax, and upper arms (Fig. 18.5) [2, 7, 15, 22, 28, 32, 41–43, 46, 53, 63]. It is rare to find the eruption above the breasts, on the hands and feet, or, like HG, involving the face [2, 43, 56]. Dyshidrosis-like lesions on the extremities are unusual [45]. Mucosal lesions have not been described [2], and excoriations are infrequent [63].

Occasionally, the urticarial papules and plaques may be so edematous that the lesions resemble papulovesicles [43]. This diverse morphology of papules, plaques, excoriations, target lesions, polycystic erythema, and vesicles led Holmes and Black [32] to classify the eruption as PEP. They reported vesicular lesions in 44% of cases [33]. In a small number of cases, small bullae may be seen as a result of coalescing vesicles [21]; however, their presence should raise clinical suspicion for HG [22, 56].

Fig. 18.1 Pruritic urticarial papules and plaques of pregnancy (PUPPP). Papular edematous erythemic lesions arranged in a herpetiform pattern. Vesicles are not seen. Note the free zone around the umbilicus

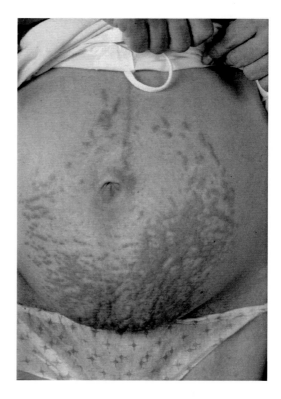

Fig. 18.2 PUPPP. Typical lesions. Note the lesions inside the striae distensae

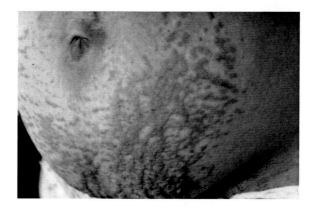

Owing to the variable clinical morphology of PUPPP, Aronson et al. [7] divided the clinical features into three types: type I, for the most part urticarial papules and plaques; type II, nonurticarial erythema, papules, or vesicles; and type III, a combination of the two forms. It should be noted, however, that generally the eruption is morphologically uniform

18

Fig. 18.3 PUPPP. Typical urticarial rash

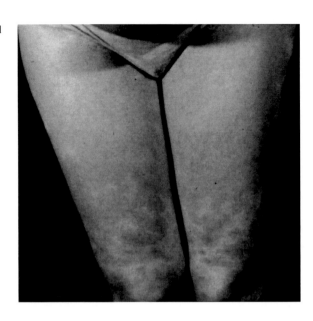

Fig. 18.4 PUPPP. Typical rash on the abdomen. Note the free zone around the umbilicus and lesions inside the striae distensae

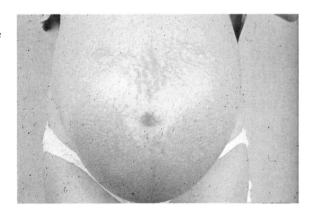

for a given patient [43]. Since the type of PUPPP has no impact on prognosis or treatment, this subclassification seems unnecessary.

Patients report extreme pruritus, often disturbing daily activities and sleep [43], but there is no systemic toxicity [63]. The duration of the symptoms is usually brief, with a mean duration of 6 weeks [2], Along with the pruritus, most eruptions clear within days to 2 weeks of delivery [15, 20, 53]; however, some fade away just before delivery [15]. In the majority of cases, as the eruption resolves, a fine scaling on the affected areas, quite similar to an eczematous appearance, may develop [11, 21]. It is rare to have postpartum onset or flare of this eruption [43].

Fig. 18.5 Areas of involvement of PUPPP

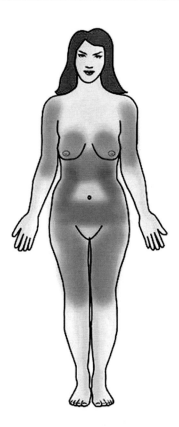

It is generally a disease of the first pregnancy (75–85%), but first onset after multiple normal gestations has been noted, especially in association with large-for-dates babies or multiple pregnancies (twins or triplets) [1, 2, 56, 64]. Recurrence in subsequent pregnancies is rare, unless it is associated with twin or multiple pregnancies, but one group has noted recurrence in up to 50% of cases [2, 34]. Oral contraceptive agents have not been found to be connected to the development of PUPPP [24]. In exceptional cases, familial occurrence was reported [62].

18.5
Laboratory Findings

Laboratory test findings are normal, and may help only to exclude concurrent problems [26, 56]. Complete blood count, findings of liver function tests, urinary human chorionic gonadotropin levels, findings of serologic tests for syphilis, and serum levels of estrogen and progesterone were normal in all reported cases [1, 42, 53, 54, 56, 60]. A decrease in the level of circulatory immune complexes during the acute phase of PUPPP has been reported [38], but the importance of this finding is unclear.

18.6
Histopathology

Histologic findings are not specific, vary according to the clinical stage of the eruption, and there are many similarities with the early, prebullous phase of HG [2, 15, 32, 42, 46]. Two patterns of skin participation have been described. A superficial type consists of perivascular lymphohistiocytic infiltration associated with some edema of the papillary dermis. In some patients the epidermis reveals focal spongiosis, mild acanthosis, patchy parakeratosis, exocytosis of eosinophils, and hyperkeratosis [2, 16, 27, 32, 39, 42, 46, 53]. A deeper pattern is characterized by perivascular and interstitial infiltrates in the mid-dermis, where the lymphocytes and histiocytes are admixed with some eosinophils [42, 53, 56]. The number of eosinophils may be striking, and differentiation from the early, prebullous phase of HG can be difficult [32, 39, 42, 46]. The papillary dermis is edematous, which may lead to subepidermal vesicle formation, but the epidermis is uninvolved [2, 42, 53]. There is no leukocytoclastic vasculitis [16, 42].

Direct immunofluorescence testing was performed on normal and lesional skin and was constantly negative; however, there have been some ambivalent direct immunofluorescence findings, such as minimal linear or granular C3 deposition along the basement membrane zone (BMZ), fibrin in the dermis, antiepidermal cell surface antibodies in one case, and one case where C3 deposition was found in one dermal vessel wall [3, 4, 7, 42, 53, 59, 64]. Direct immunofluorescence testing can also rarely show a speckled band of IgM deposition along the BMZ [2]. Zurn et al. [66] described five patients with PUPPP who had circulating anti-BMZ antibodies of IgM isotype. The specificity of this observation has been debated [12, 31].

Indirect immunofluorescence tests were negative [57]. Immunoelectron microscopy is also regularly negative. Direct immunofluorescence testing provides the best means of distinguishing this disorder from HG, where immunofluorescence testing is essentially positive, should there be any diagnostic doubt [37, 61].

18.7
Physiopathology

The cause of this eruption is unknown [43], and there has been much speculation about the factors that contribute to its pathogenesis [12]. The nonspecific histologic picture and the negative laboratory workup add little to our understanding of the disease [53]. Evidence for an immunologic basis is lacking [63]. Histocompatibility antigen (HLA) determinations in patients with PUPPP are no different than in the general population and it does not appear to be associated with autoimmune disorders [10, 21, 24, 64]. The search for circulating immune complexes and deposition of immunoreactants in the skin was unrewarding in the majority of patients [10, 38, 64]. It has no association with preeclampsia or HG [2, 39].

The condition has been related to abnormal weight gains in the mother and the newborn and to twin pregnancies (13 of 114 cases, one case of triplets) [14, 22, 23]. This observation in addition to the fact that the disorder occurs predominantly in primigravidas with prominent striae in the third trimester led to the hypothesis that rapid, late, excessive abdominal distension resulting in collagen and elastic fiber damage in striae, with subsequent conversion of nonantigenic molecules to antigenic ones, may act as a trigger for the inflammatory skin changes [8, 10, 11, 14, 23, 47, 48, 56]. It is interesting to note that Bourne [13] made similar observations in his original series of patients with so-called toxemic rash of pregnancy in 1962.

The association with maternal or fetal weight gain has been questioned [51, 61], but a meta-analysis performed by Kroumpouzos and Cohen [40] in 2003 found 29 multiple gestation pregnancies in 282 PUPPP cases (11.7%). This prevalence was at least tenfold higher than the prevalence of multiple gestations in the USA (1%) [30]. The association of PUPPP with multiple gestation was further supported by the study of Elling et al. [25], which reported a prevalence of 7.89 PUPPP cases out of 200 multiple-gestation pregnancies, compared with one PUPPP case out of 200 singleton pregnancies [25].

The clinical presentation suggests some form of hypersensitivity reaction [53], and an association of 11% of patients with PUPPP with asthma was found [7]. Several studies indicate the activation of the skin immune system to maternal and/or fetal antigens [6, 18, 58]. Immunohistochemical studies showed an infiltrate that is composed mainly of T-helper lymphocytes [18, 58], and immunohistologic profiling of these activated T cells in the dermis and of epidermal Langerhans cells suggests a delayed hypersensitivity reaction to an unknown antigen [40].

Fetal causes may contribute to the origin of PUPPP, as it has been reported to be more common with male fetuses, with a male-to-female ratio of 2:1 in the outcome in affected women [61]. Arcatingi et al. [6] in 1998 reported ten pregnant patients who all had a male fetus and PUPPP. This association was confirmed recently in a retrospective case-control study [49]; Regnier et al. [49] showed that 64.5% of the women in the PEP group had male fetuses compared with 48.4% in the control group. Male DNA was detected at the dermoepidermal junction in six of the ten patients. Pregnancy is associated with peripheral blood chimerism, predominantly during the third trimester. This fact in addition to increased abdominal stretching, which increases vascular permeability, may assist the migration of chimeric cells into the maternal skin [40], causing eruptions in susceptible individuals [44, 55]. A paternal factor hypothetically generated or expressed by the fetal portion of the placenta has been invoked as the cause of PUPPP in two families with unusual conjugal patterns [62].

The author and his colleagues [36] speculated that during the aging of the placenta in the third trimester a substance is released into the maternal circulation that may trigger fibroblast proliferation. This assumption was based on the histologic appearance of multiple dermal fibroblasts with no deposition of mucin (Fig. 18.6). This hypothesis has not been supported by other studies [40].

No reliable hormonal abnormalities have been found [5, 10, 21], but the hormonal contribution is not excluded, as one patient had persistent pruritus during 2 months of breast-feeding, followed by flares of pruritus localized to the hands during nine successive

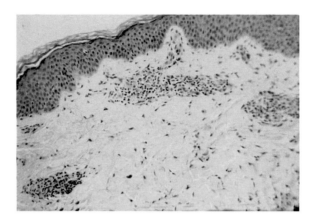

Fig. 18.6 PUPPP. Hematoxylin and eosin stain. Perivascular lymphocytic infiltrate in the upper dermis. Many fibroblasts are scattered in the dermis

menstrual periods [42, 53]. Another patient developed two transient episodes of hives with breast-feeding [42, 53]. Multiple gestations, which are presumably interconnected to PUPPP, are associated with higher estrogen and progesterone levels [17]. In addition, progesterone has been shown to worsen the inflammatory process at the tissue level. Corresponding to this, in cultures of human keratinocytes, lesional epidermis of PUPPP has shown amplified progesterone receptor expression by immunoreactivity and reverse transcriptase polymerase chain reaction. Nonlesional epidermis, however, has not revealed any progesterone receptor positivity [35].

Other hormonal factors claimed to take part in the functional changes are suggested by a prospective study of 44 cases of PUPPP, which showed low serum cortisol levels, compared with those of normal control pregnant women [61].

18.8
Diagnosis

Drug rashes must remain highly suspect [56]. Fortunately, pregnancy is generally a time of restricted drug use [56]. In addition, drug eruption can be ruled out by an appropriate history [63]. Toxic erythemas of viral origin are usually apparent within the context of associated symptoms [56]. The most important differential is the rare urticarial form of HG [56]. The only secure way to exclude this is by immunofluorescence studies [56].

PUPPP is distinguished from pruritic folliculitis of pregnancy on the basis of the follicular character of the lesions and histopathologic features in pruritic folliculitis of pregnancy

[39, 65]. Prurigo of pregnancy begins earlier in pregnancy, lacks urticarial lesions, persists throughout pregnancy, and may recur with subsequent pregnancies [39, 46]. The differentiation between PUPPP and intrahepatic cholestasis of pregnancy (ICP) is possible by comprehensive clinical history, absence of primary skin lesions in ICP, serology, and recurrence in subsequent pregnancies of ICP [39, 50] Erythema multiforme is another condition which may be indistinguishable from PUPPP [42, 53].

18.9
Treatment

Treatment of PUPPP depends on the severity of the symptoms. It should include reassurance about the self-limited, benign nature of the disease in spite of the severe pruritus, and symptomatic treatment is usually sufficient. This can be in the form of emollients, antipruritic topical medications (menthol, doxepin), and systemic antihistamines, such as chlorpheniramine, as an antipruritic agent [2, 15, 43, 56].

Although their use is not recommended, moderately potent topical corticosteroid creams may be needed by some patients to get relief from pruritus [42, 53, 56, 63]. Topical applications may be tapered according to symptomatic control [43], and generally patients may stop using topical steroids in time for delivery [43]. Difficult cases, with distressing pruritus, can be safely managed with a tapering regimen of orally administered prednisone starting with 30–40 mg/day for 7–14 days [2, 63]. UVB therapy was reported to be successful in treating several patients with PUPPP [39].

A severe case of PUPPP, unresponsive to therapy, was dramatically improved within 2 h after cesarean section delivery [9]. This modality of treatment has been debated [19].

18.10
Prognosis

There is no known association between PUPPP and other cutaneous or systemic diseases [56]. No fetal or maternal complications have been reported, but pruritus may be severe and intractable [39]. One neonate was described by Ahmed and Kaplan to have an eruption clinically and histologically resembling PUPPP that cleared spontaneously [60, 63]. The babies tend to be larger than normal [23], and the number of twin or multiple pregnancies in PUPPP appears to be significantly increased [49, 61]. An unusually high sex ratio (increased number of male fetuses) has been reported [49, 61]. A recent report by Regnier et al. [49] showed that PEP was significantly associated with cesarean section (40%) compared with controls (13.1%). The two most common indications for cesarean section in this study were inadequate progression of labor and breech presentation.

18

Summary

› Pruritic urticarial papules and plaques of pregnancy (PUPPP) is most common dermatosis of pregnancy, with an incidence of one in 120–300 pregnancies.
› It typically presents during the third trimester in primigravidas, and there is increased incidence with multiple pregnancies and with maternal and fetal weight gain.
› It has variable presentation, but usually appears as pruritic erythematous papules and plaques on the striae in the lower abdomen, sparing the umbilicus. Subsequently the rash spreads to the trunk and proximal extremities.
› Laboratory test findings are classically normal.
› The histopathologic characteristics are nonspecific, showing perivascular infiltration and spongiosis in the epidermis.
› It is important to differentiate PUPPP from herpes gestationis. The best method is by immunofluorescence studies.
› The cause is unknown, but a potential role of abdominal wall distension as a trigger for inflammation has been hypothesized.
› Treatment is usually symptomatic, but sometimes systemic steroids may be needed.
› Prognosis is excellent for both mother and fetus. Cesarean sections may be more common. Recurrences are rare.

References

1. Ahmed AR, Kaplan R (1981) Pruritic urticarial papules and plaques of pregnancy. J Am Acad Dermatol 4:679–681
2. Al-Fares SI, Jones SV, Black MM (2001) The specific dermatoses of pregnancy: a re-appraisal. J Eur Acad Dermatol Venereol 15:197–206
3. Alcalay J, David M, Sandbank M (1986) Facial involvement in pruritic urticarial papules and plaques of pregnancy. J Am Acad Dermatol 15:1048
4. Alcalay J, Ingber A, David M et al (1987) Pruritic urticarial papules and plaques of pregnancy. A review of 21 cases. J Reprod Med 32:315–316
5. Alcalay J, Ingber A, Kafri B et al (1988) Hormonal evaluation and autoimmune background in pruritic urticarial papules and plaques of pregnancy. Am J Obstet Gynecol 158:417–420
6. Aractingi S, Berkane N, Bertheau P et al (1998) Fetal DNA in skin of polymorphic eruptions of pregnancy. Lancet 352:1898–1901
7. Aronson IK, Bond S, Fiedler VC et al (1998) Pruritic urticarial papules and plaques of pregnancy: clinical and immunopathologic observations in 57 patients. J Am Acad Dermatol 39:933–939
8. Beckett MA, Goldberg NS (1991) Pruritic urticarial plaques and papules of pregnancy and skin distention. Arch Dermatol 127:125–126
9. Beltrani VP, Beltrani VS (1992) Pruritic urticarial papules and plaques of pregnancy: a severe case requiring early delivery for relief of symptoms. J Am Acad Dermatol 26:266–267
10. Black M, Stephens C (1989) The specific dermatoses of pregnancy: the British perspective. Adv Dermatol 7:105–127

11. Black MM (1997) Progress and new directions in the investigation of the specific dermatoses of pregnancy. Keio J Med 46:40–41
12. Borradori L, Saurat JH (1994) Specific dermatoses of pregnancy. Toward a comprehensive view? Arch Dermatol 130:778–780
13. Bourne G (1962) Toxaemic rash of pregnancy. Proc R Soc Med 55:462–464
14. Bunker CB, Erskine K, Rustin MH et al (1990) Severe polymorphic eruption of pregnancy occurring in twin pregnancies. Clin Exp Dermatol 15:228–231
15. Callen JP (1984) Pregnancy's effects on the skin. Common and uncommon changes. Postgrad Med 75:138–145
16. Callen JP, Hanno R (1981) Pruritic urticarial papules and plaques of pregnancy (PUPPP). A clinicopathologic study. J Am Acad Dermatol 5:401–405
17. Campbell DM (1986) Maternal adaptation in twin pregnancy. Semin Perinatol 10:14–18
18. Carli P, Tarocchi S, Mello G et al (1994) Skin immune system activation in pruritic urticarial papules and plaques of pregnancy. Int J Dermatol 33:884–885
19. Carruthers A (1993) Pruritic urticarial papules and plaques of pregnancy. J Am Acad Dermatol 29:125
20. Catanzarite V, Quirk JG Jr (1990) Papular dermatoses of pregnancy. Clin Obstet Gynecol 33:754–758
21. Charles-Holmes R (1989) Polymorphic eruption of pregnancy. Semin Dermatol 8:18–22
22. Cohen LM (1998) Dermatoses of pregnancy. West J Med 169:223–224
23. Cohen LM, Capeless EL, Krusinski PA et al (1989) Pruritic urticarial papules and plaques of pregnancy and its relationship to maternal-fetal weight gain and twin pregnancy. Arch Dermatol 125:1534–1536
24. Dacus JV (1990) Pruritus in pregnancy. Clin Obstet Gynecol 33:738–745
25. Elling SV, McKenna P, Powell FC (2000) Pruritic urticarial papules and plaques of pregnancy in twin and triplet pregnancies. J Eur Acad Dermatol Venereol 14:378–381
26. Errickson CV, Matus NR (1994) Skin disorders of pregnancy. Am Fam Physician 49:605–610
27. Eudy SF, Baker GF (1990) Dermatopathology for the obstetrician. Clin Obstet Gynecol 33:728–737
28. Fox GN (1986) Pruritic urticarial papules and plaques of pregnancy. Am Fam Physician 34:191–195
29. Fuhrman L (2000) Common dermatoses of pregnancy. J Perinat Neonatal Nurs 14:1–16
30. Hays PM, Smeltzer JS (1986) Multiple gestation. Clin Obstet Gynecol 29:264–285
31. Helm TN, Valenzuela R (1992) Continuous dermoepidermal junction IgM detected by direct immunofluorescence: a report of nine cases. J Am Acad Dermatol 26:203–206
32. Holmes RC, Black MM (1982) The specific dermatoses of pregnancy: a reappraisal with special emphasis on a proposed simplified clinical classification. Clin Exp Dermatol 7:65–73
33. Holmes RC, Black MM (1983) The specific dermatoses of pregnancy. J Am Acad Dermatol 8:405–412
34. Holmes RC, Black MM, Dann J et al (1982) A comparative study of toxic erythema of pregnancy and herpes gestationis. Br J Dermatol 106:499–510
35. Im S, Lee ES, Kim W et al (2000) Expression of progesterone receptor in human keratinocytes. J Korean Med Sci 15:647–654
36. Ingber A, Alcalay J, Sandbank M (1988) Multiple dermal fibroblasts in patients with pruritic urticarial papules and plaques of pregnancy. A clue to the etiology? Med Hypotheses 26:11–12
37. Jurecka W, Holmes RC, Black MM et al (1983) An immunoelectron microscopy study of the relationship between herpes gestationis and polymorphic eruption of pregnancy. Br J Dermatol 108:147–151

38. Kasp-Grochowska E, Beck J, Holmes RC et al (1984) The role of circulating immune complexes in the aetiology of polymorphic eruption of pregnancy. Arch Dermatol Res 276:71–73
39. Kroumpouzos G, Cohen LM (2001) Dermatoses of pregnancy. J Am Acad Dermatol 45:1–19; quiz 19–22
40. Kroumpouzos G, Cohen LM (2003) Specific dermatoses of pregnancy: an evidence-based systematic review. Am J Obstet Gynecol 188:1083–1092
41. Lawley TJ, Stingl G, Katz SI (1978) Fetal and maternal risk factors in herpes gestationis. Arch Dermatol 114:552–555
42. Lawley TJ, Hertz KC, Wade TR et al (1979) Pruritic urticarial papules and plaques of pregnancy. JAMA 241:1696–1699
43. Murray JC (1990) Pregnancy and the skin. Dermatol Clin 8:327–334
44. Nelson JL, Furst DE, Maloney S et al (1998) Microchimerism and HLA-compatible relationships of pregnancy in scleroderma. Lancet 351:559–562
45. Normand F, Armingaud P, Esteve E (2001) Dyshidrosis and acral purpura during polymorphic dermatitis in pregnancy: 2 cases. Ann Dermatol Venereol 128:531–533
46. Nurse DS (1968) Prurigo of pregnancy. Australas J Dermatol 9:258–267
47. Pauwels C, Bucaille-Fleury L, Recanati G (1994) Pruritic urticarial papules and plaques of pregnancy: relationship to maternal weight gain and twin or triplet pregnancies. Arch Dermatol 130:801–802
48. Powell FC (1992) Parity, polypregnancy, paternity, and PUPPP. Arch Dermatol 128:1551
49. Regnier S, Fermand V, Levy P et al (2008) A case-control study of polymorphic eruption of pregnancy. J Am Acad Dermatol 58:63–67
50. Reyes H (1982) The enigma of intrahepatic cholestasis of pregnancy: lessons from Chile. Hepatology 2:87–96
51. Roger D, Vaillant L, Lorette G (1990) Pruritic urticarial papules and plaques of pregnancy are not related to maternal or fetal weight gain. Arch Dermatol 126:1517
52. Roger D, Vaillant L, Fignon A et al (1994) Specific pruritic diseases of pregnancy. A prospective study of 3192 pregnant women. Arch Dermatol 130:734–739
53. Sasseville D, Wilkinson RD, Schnader JY (1981) Dermatoses of pregnancy. Int J Dermatol 20:223–241
54. Schwartz RA, Hansen RC, Lynch PJ (1981) Pruritic urticarial papules and plaques of pregnancy. Cutis 27:425–426, 432
55. Sherard GB 3rd, Atkinson SM Jr (2001) Focus on primary care: pruritic dermatological conditions in pregnancy. Obstet Gynecol Surv 56:427–432
56. Shornick JK (1998) Dermatoses of pregnancy. Semin Cutan Med Surg 17:172–181
57. Sodhi VK, Sausker WF (1988) Dermatoses of pregnancy. Am Fam Physician 37:131–138
58. Tarocchi S, Carli P, Caproni M et al (1997) Polymorphic eruption of pregnancy. Int J Dermatol 36:448–450
59. Trattner A, Ingber A, Sandbank M (1991) Antiepidermal cell surface antibodies in a patient with pruritic urticarial papules and plaques of pregnancy. J Am Acad Dermatol 24:306–308
60. Uhlin SR (1981) Pruritic urticarial papules and plaques of pregnancy. Involvement in mother and infant. Arch Dermatol 117:238–239
61. Vaughan Jones SA, Hern S, Nelson-Piercy C et al (1999) A prospective study of 200 women with dermatoses of pregnancy correlating clinical findings with hormonal and immunopathological profiles. Br J Dermatol 141:71–81
62. Weiss R, Hull P (1992) Familial occurrence of pruritic urticarial papules and plaques of pregnancy. J Am Acad Dermatol 26:715–717
63. Winton GB, Lewis CW (1982) Dermatoses of pregnancy. J Am Acad Dermatol 6:977–998

64. Yancey KB, Hall RP, Lawley TJ (1984) Pruritic urticarial papules and plaques of pregnancy. Clinical experience in twenty-five patients. J Am Acad Dermatol 10:473–480
65. Zoberman E, Farmer ER (1981) Pruritic folliculitis of pregnancy. Arch Dermatol 117:20–22
66. Zurn A, Celebi CR, Bernard P et al (1992) A prospective immunofluorescence study of 111 cases of pruritic dermatoses of pregnancy: IgM anti-basement membrane zone antibodies as a novel finding. Br J Dermatol 126:474–478

Index

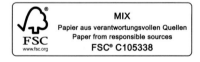
Printed by Books on Demand, Germany